MEDICINE AND NURSING

Professions in a
Changing Health Service

Sylvia Walby and June Greenwell
with
Lesley Mackay and Keith Soothill

SAGE Publications

London • Thousand Oaks • New Delhi

First published 1994

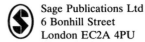 Sage Publications Ltd
6 Bonhill Street
London EC2A 4PU

SAGE Publications Inc
2455 Teller Road
Thousand Oaks, California 91320

SAGE Publications India Pvt Ltd
32, M-Block Market
Greater Kailash – I
New Delhi 110 048

British Library Cataloguing in Publication data

A catalogue record for this book is available from the
British Library

ISBN 0 8039 8741 2
ISBN 0 8039 8742 0 (pbk)

Library of Congress catalog card number 94–067258

Typeset by Photoprint, Torquay, Devon
Printed in Great Britain by Biddles Ltd, Guildford, Surrey

MEDICINE AND NURSING

Contents

List of Figures and Tables

Acknowledgements

In the process of writing the book we have drawn on several sources of information. A section of the book draws on the findings of a study of interprofessional relations of medical and nursing staff in hospitals. We are pleased to acknowledge the generosity of the doctors, nurses and other hospital staff we interviewed for giving their time so freely to this study. We are sorry we can name neither the individuals who have helped, nor the hospitals where interviews took place, but this is essential in order to maintain the confidentiality of our respondents. We are, of course, entirely responsible for the arguments in this book. We wish to thank the ESRC for grant number R000 23 1394 which funded this research; and the individuals who helped to make the research possible. We would like to thank Brian Francis of Lancaster University Centre for Applied Statistics for his help in analysing the statistics and revealing for us the information contained within them. We also wish to thank the officers and members of Lancaster CHC who over several years have informed our understanding of the health service.

1

Introduction

In the past decade the organisation of work has changed. The pursuit of excellence is a common theme. Excellence requires managers to focus on the people who produce the product, and the people who consume the goods. Innovative, collaborative, loosely managed teams who are close to the customer are the ideal 'unit of production'.

In the health service, professional workers produce a significant part of the 'product'. They are close to the customer, they often have to work in teams, and they make independent, autonomous, decisions. Yet the health professions have been under attack. They are increasingly being 'managed', and in the process losing the autonomy that at one time characterised their activity.

Something is wrong. If the autonomous team is the ideal, why are autonomous teams of professionals so urgently needing to be managed? Is 'new wave' management an inappropriate approach to public services that are dominated by professionals, or are professions self-interested organisations, lacking a proper focus on their customers, and refusing to collaborate in the interest of the people they serve?

We look for answers to these questions by examining in detail the collaborative work of doctors and nurses in one area of professional work: acute hospital wards. Highly trained, knowledge-based, autonomous workers are going to be typical of the future, according to many theorists of post-Fordist, post-industrial and post-capitalist society (Bell, 1973; Drucker, 1993; Piore and Sabel, 1984). Doctors and nurses are leading examples of such workers. The relationship between them is the empirical core of this book; the debate on employment change its theoretical focus.

Health work has been at the cutting edge of a politically inspired attempt to restructure working practices in Britain over the past decade. Attempts at creating markets, giving priority to consumers over producers, introducing new forms of management and cost containment, have turned the health service into a laboratory of experimentation in changing working practices. The health service is an important area of employment, both because of its size (the National Health Service is the largest employer in the UK) and because of its work practices, which simultaneously combine old classic forms with those at the forefront of change. Today, health work is being reorganised to reflect the new political priorities of the 1990s, though the organisation of key workers into professions represents a pre-industrial form of work organisation. New issues interact with old lines of conflict in the health professions. We look at the lines of professional interaction in the context of these new changes.

Health work is more typical of contemporary forms of work than the conventional sociological examples of car workers on the factory floor. Manufacturing work has been the basis of most sociology of work, as it has for much management theory. Peters and Austin (1986), reflecting on the poor achievement of American public sector organisations, sees the adoption of industrial management systems as the key factor in their poor track record: 'Much of the reason is surely that their managers adopted, with sadly little reflection, the management techniques that were so highly praised in the industrial sector' (1986: xviii). Yet in the 1990s most work is in services. The sorts of jobs which have formed the basis of most sociological and management theorising have been almost entirely eliminated in the UK. This study of work issues in health is more typical of employment in general than the usual study.

The dominant theme in the contemporary sociology of the professions focuses on professionalisation as a collective strategy to enhance the rewards and power of members of the profession. The professionalisation of both medicine and nursing is considered primarily as a self-seeking strategy by groups of workers. Professionalisation strategies have been considered in the context of wider social structures such as those of class and, more recently, gender (Elston, 1991; Moran and Wood, 1993; Witz, 1992). The traditional agenda has focused on relations between producers, on hierarchies at work between bosses and workers, or, in the case of health, between bureaucrats and professionals.

A more recent emphasis is that on the relations between producers and consumers. This stems from a critique of the welfare state which suggests that it is run for its workers rather than for its clients. This agenda emerged on the Left as a critique of faceless bureaucrats who treated clients without dignity. Its strongest articulation has come from the Right in its espousal of the rights of individual consumers over collectively organised producers. Changes in NHS cultural values stress the significance of the patient as a 'consumer', in a way that relates to changing theoretical conceptualisations.

Health work is again more typical of British 'industry' than that usually studied because of its gender composition, with women comprising about half the workforce. Most sociology of work has been based on men's work and men's relationships with other men at work. Yet in the 1990s women form very nearly half the workforce, and the relationship between the sexes at work is crucial. The segregation of the sexes is a central feature of work organisation. The analysis of gender in the workplace is not merely one of simple hierarchy, sometimes suggested in the literature, but of complex cross-cutting forms of difference and subordination. What happens to women workers, who are highly trained and qualified, in their relationship to male workers?

One aspect of health work which is atypical makes it even more important – it is growing. The demand for health care increases with the demographic shift in the age structure of the population – old people want and need more health care – and as improvements in medical technology make more interventions possible. The current crisis in health work is at least partly due to the clash between this increased demand for health care and a government committed to the limitation of public expenditure, though the issue of cost containment in health care is a widespread concern of governments throughout the Western world. Theories of employment, management and professionalisation need revision to be consistent with these transformations. Recent theorisations of post-Fordism are the most interesting attempts to encompass the changes.

Fordism and health services

Hospitals have organisational structures that relate directly to Fordist and post-Fordist ideas. When he established his car factory, Henry Ford lent his name to a dynamic of change leading to the simplification of jobs that could be done by cheaper and less skilled labour. Work is organised on a production line, if possible, with each worker contributing one small part to the whole process. Applied to health such a thesis would predict the constant subdivision of medical tasks so that they could be carried out by workers who could be trained more narrowly for shorter periods, and paid less, with more exactly defined duties carefully supervised by managers. Should each care assistant or nurse be highly specialised and trained only to undertake a narrow focus of tasks, with the patient serviced by mobile teams of staff? Similarly, should doctors and hospitals specialise in providing particular forms of surgery, so as to achieve higher quality mass production of surgical operations? If cataract operations can be conducted *en masse*, effectively and cheaply, by a mobile team of professionals, why maintain a myriad of small eye surgery units in district hospitals each performing some cataract work? Could a skill-mix of fewer professionals and more narrowly trained support workers provide as good or better care, with some cost benefits? Henry Ford would be at ease with such an argument.

Fordism has sometimes been considered to have had an effect not only on the immediate labour process via a Taylorist style of management but on a number of related areas as well. For instance, Edwards (1979) has argued that the organisation of the worker developed to parallel that of the employer, with the growth of mass trade unionism. In some respects, and from a number of ostensibly quite contrary theoretical perspectives, this is a compelling thesis – factories got bigger, mainstream economists argued, in order to take advantage of economies of scale. Work was deskilled, Marxist social scientists asserted, so that employers could employ cheaper labour and control it more effectively (Braverman, 1974; but see Elger, 1979, Friedman, 1977; Wood, 1989).

Post-Fordism

Post-Fordist theorists argue that there is currently a major transition in Western societies away from Fordist principles of organisation. The new phase is marked by flexible working practices in which employers use new technology to make varied products which can be sold more effectively to a market which has become highly differentiated, so replacing Fordism with its mass production and mass consumption. New technology means that economies of scale no longer apply. We could cross a 'second industrial divide' into an era of product differentiation and enriched jobs (Piore and Sabel, 1984). This optimistic vision of a post-Fordist society includes jobs which are enskilled as a result of the leaving behind of the monotony of mass production. Niche markets replace the mass markets of Fordism. No longer is every motor car black, but there is a choice not only of colour, but also of engine size, sun roof, electric windows, in-car stereo and so on.

The strength of the post-Fordist thesis is its attempt to grasp and theorise an awareness of the power of the new technology and that work practices, not only the actual labour, but also the form of the labour contract, are not static, but constantly undergoing change. It catches the sense that mass assembly lines are not a civilised way to work and embodies a desire to do better, tempered by a realisation of the limits of a hierarchically driven social system. There are, though, numerous difficulties in transferring to a nation-wide system of state-funded health provision an organisational model of production based on the notion of niche marketing. The absence of a market in health care, a high value placed on equity of provision and the absence of consumers empowered to pay for services are pertinent factors. Perhaps most significant is the nature of NHS work as an emergency service. Hip replacement operations may be a suitable area for niche marketing, as the development of the private hospital sector has suggested, but creating a niche market in hip operations at one hospital could threaten the staffing and financial viability of the accident and emergency service at another hospital, so finely balanced are the budgets for services. Niche marketing and equitable provision of emergency health care coexist uneasily. Nevertheless, some of the changes in NHS organisation are explicable in terms of a commitment to a post-Fordist model of health care.

The optimistic scenario of Piore and Sabel (1984), in which all jobs can be enriched, contrasts with the more pessimistic version of Atkinson (1986). Flexibility is not merely of the 'functional' kind where workers are enskilled, but also 'numerical' where a peripheral workforce bears the brunt of fluctuations in the demand for labour. The periphery is distanced from the core of the company by a range of devices including sub-contracting, temporary contracts and part-time working (see Atkinson, 1986; Bagguley et al., 1990).

Just as Fordism exists in hospitals, so do the variations of post-Fordism. A hospital consultant, a primary nurse and a Nissan car worker have the common features of skill, some autonomy in decision making, and responsiveness to the demands of the customer. The development of NHS Trust hospitals theoretically gives Trust Boards and their managers a similar autonomy, in order to unite the skilled professional and his or her Trust employer in a mutual commitment to high-quality, patient-responsive care. Manager and professionals unite in the optimistic variant of post-Fordism, both looking to the customer to determine their priorities, and it is these elements of post-Fordism that have influenced the NHS reforms. Whether the Trusts have actually acquired a significant degree of autonomy, and whether they have used their autonomy to serve customer rather than institutional goals, is a matter of some controversy.

Examples of the less optimistic variant of post-Fordism are also present. Contracting out of services for ancillary staff has been normal practice for some time, and some paramedical services such as laboratory work have been considered as suitable for contracting out. The development of GP budget holding and NHS Trust hospitals means that service providers will make decisions that they think best suit their needs. This is likely to increase the tendency to form a divide between core and peripheral service units, as suppliers offer to individual GPs and Trusts services that do not have to carry the costs of wider public health service obligations. It is a process similar to the sub-contracting of work to peripheral contractors that is a feature of post-Fordist production. Hospitals have used a system of core and peripheral nursing staff for many years, with the employment of bank and agency nurses to deal with variations in workload. The emphasis here is on meeting service needs in a flexible way, rather than the casualisation of employment, but it has given nurse managers considerable experience in the flexible employment of staff in a post-Fordist manner.

While the more global forms of post-Fordist theory are over-ambitious, none the less, the theory is a powerful tool for the analysis of the differences between specific areas of work. Both Fordist and post-Fordist modes of organisation can and do coexist, despite the tensions between them. The grading system for nurses, the move to have tighter contracts for medical consultants, and discussions about using narrowly trained care workers to take over nursing tasks, are all examples of a Fordist approach to hospital organisation. Primary nursing and traditional medical autonomy both fit into the positive variant of post-Fordism.

Professions and post-Fordism

The debate on post-Fordism addresses the questions of whether there are general principles by which work can be more efficiently organised and whether this is necessarily at the expense of the workers' conditions of employment. There is postulated a major divergence between two widely different logics of work organisation. One, represented in Fordism, is that of ever tighter and more detailed control over workers by bosses, in order to improve the level of work output. The second, represented in post-Fordism, relies upon the self-motivation of a skilled worker engaged in meaningful activity to do his or her best at work. The first considers that greater control over the worker is the way to greater output, the second more worker autonomy. Whether there has been a movement from a Fordist logic of work organisation to a post-Fordist one is a major focus of the discussion of the work of doctors and nurses in this book. It considers how detailed changes in employment practices in the health service might be understood in the wider context of the debate on post-Fordism.

The traditional organisation of work within the professions shares some striking similarities with that described as post-Fordist, and there are some good theoretical reasons why there should be such similarities. Health work is an area where significant numbers of workers have high levels of education, and is a service sector industry with a focus on work with people. The presumption here is that highly skilled workers need greater autonomy to carry out their work effectively than those who have less skill. These are also the features of the cutting edge industries of post-Fordism.

However, there are some exceptions and some important variations in the extent to which skilled workers have more autonomy than less-skilled workers. First, there is the contentious impact of some aspects of the reforms of the NHS. If one aim of the reforms was to provide innovative and autonomous work teams, then the impact of some change has been contradictory, in that there is a reduction in the autonomy of consultants and GPs. The work of doctors is increasingly scrutinised, so that consultants are losing some autonomy to other medical colleagues through medical audit, and all consultants are having to respond to the discipline of service contracts. Many GPs have lost ease of referral to specialist hospitals through a requirement to either conform to contractual arrangements, or to have extra-contractual referrals timetabled to comply with the exigencies of health authority budgets. Secondly, there are questions as to whether nursing is organised on as autonomous a basis as might be expected given the level of skill and training involved.

There is no direct market relationship between the health professional (as producer) and the patient (as consumer), though there is a service relationship that appears to be valued. Where patients' wishes have been studied, there is a preference for trusting the doctor, rather than assessing the quality of the medical services provided (Illman, 1991, Lupton et al., 1991). In so far as a market has been introduced in the NHS it is not between the producer and the consumer/patient, but between producers. Managers and professionals can and do seek to obtain the views of patients as users of services, but are able to ignore them. There is no mechanism to compel either manager or professional to give priority to consumer preferences. A key factor is that the UK health market is a market for rationed services. However responsive, flexible and committed they may be, hospital staff can only provide NHS services that their district health authority or GP can afford to buy. Optimistic theorisations of post-Fordist tendencies in health care ignore limitations to the job-enrichment of autonomous skilled work in public services dominated by tightly constrained budgets.

Post-Fordism has been used to capture within a single theory changes that are encompassing the whole of society, as in the regulation school of Aglietta (1987) and Jessop (1991), while other writers focus on relations in employment (Atkinson, 1986). The development of new forms of management theory and practice, sometimes known as 'new wave management', but also 'human resource management' (see Clarke et al., 1994), has much in common with post-Fordist conceptualisation, but is focused on the management of organisations. Does 'new wave' management usefully explain the contradiction between simultaneously encouraging and restricting the autonomy of professional workers? Does it give a model that clarifies how the work of professionals fits within a managed and rationed health care market?

New wave management and professionals

'New wave management' has at its core a belief that workers can be more productive if they are encouraged to use all their abilities in a relatively free, rather than closely monitored, way. This is a practice which is also part of post-Fordist modes of governance, at least of core workers. Traditional management theory emphasised structures of control over the workforce, while the newer approaches emphasise the benefits of utilising workers' skills and effort by engaging their commitment and positioning them closer to markets and consumers (Peters and Waterman, 1982; Wood, 1989).

There is a tension between the new and the old forms of management in the contemporary NHS, even as they rather uneasily coexist. Further, each contains apparent contradictions. For instance, the new form of management theoretically opposes bureaucracies yet in practice introduces more, in order to run the new internal market. New wave management is a form of rhetoric as well as a set of practices, introducing changes in language as well as content. Changes supposedly primarily concerned with improving patient treatment and care can appear to be at least as concerned with cost containment. The power that energises new wave management is responsiveness to the consumer, but it is far from certain that responding to the customer can energise a system when the manager has both to act as a proxy for the customer, and remain a reliable officer responding to directives from above. Even the notion of who is the customer in the NHS is not clear. Is the consumer the patient or the purchasing authority? Is there any meaningful sense in which patients can be regarded as consumers when there is no mechanism by which they can impose their priorities as to service provision?

The organisational coordination, or management (Clarke and Newman, 1994), of many professional workers in the public sector services is changing under the pressure of the creation of markets.

The demand is for innovative staff, responsive to customer wishes, but the best practice of traditional medicine and nursing could be construed as a leading example of just the kind of highly committed, autonomous, value-led form of management that is advocated by new wave management experts (Peters, 1987; Peters and Waterman, 1982). The self-governance of some health professionals is being reshaped and to some extent restricted at precisely the moment that new management theory is advocating such autonomous styles of worker organisation. Contemporary managerialism thus contains divergent trends (Atkinson, 1986; Clarke et al., 1994), not all of which endorse such new wave thinking. These tensions within management theory and practice parallel those between Fordism and post-Fordism.

An emphasis on increasing the autonomy of workers is a central tenet of new wave management, but it is accompanied by an equal stress on the need for leadership. Leadership is portrayed as the antithesis of management. ' "Management" . . . connotes controlling and arranging and demeaning and reducing. "Leadership" connotes unleashing energy, building, freeing and growing' (Peters and Austin, 1986: xix). An emphasis on leadership fits with greater ease within a professional service perpetually required to work within tightly defined budgetary limits than does a concentration on the virtues of autonomy. Individual professional autonomy may be incompatible with a budget-led service, but if qualities of leadership are perceived as the essential factors determining service quality and output, there is theoretically no limit to the potential for inspiring workers to produce a better service. Leadership, rather than management or command, is held to be the key to greater corporate achievement.

There is, though, an essential requirement: leadership requires people to lead. In the context of the professional work of nurses and doctors in hospital, the practice of leadership could in principle be restricted to a single profession, or could involve one leader for a multi-professional team, or could fluctuate, moving from one profession to another as appropriate to the needs of patients or the characteristics of the ward. The first option is compatible with the vertical hierarchies of each profession, with nurse managers or ward sisters leading the nursing team, and consultants heading the medical team. With this model, the interprofessional ward team is a vague and leaderless abstraction.

The second option, of a single professional leader, is compatible with a model of dominant and subordinate professions, and is the pattern that appears natural to many doctors. Watkins gives an iconoclastic account of medicine that highlights this aspect of medical culture (Watkins, 1987). The third model assumes an inter-professional team in which leadership may come from different professions, and be influential across professional divides.

In emphasising the significance of leadership, new wave manage-ment by-passes traditional professional hierarchies. 'Leading' a ward team means influencing and inspiring staff from several occupational groups, some of whom have a hierarchical line management structure, and all have some accountability to senior staff within their own profession. To develop a multi-professional team necessitates forming a horizontally structured grouping of staff from vertically organised occupations. This inevitably means nego-tiating the boundaries between professions and occupations, a process particularly fraught in the context of hospital wards with a myriad of professional, technical, administrative and ancillary staff.

In this book we have chosen to examine only two of these occupations, and in only one setting: acute hospital wards. While this ignores some of the most dynamic aspects of the organisation of health care which are occurring in the move from hospital-based to community and family-based service provision, there are good reasons for choosing acute hospital wards as the setting in which to focus on doctor–nurse team working. Here there is a need to cooperate on an hour-to-hour basis and there is a wide array of different specialties, each with particular features. The hospital is still the location where junior doctors and nurses absorb the cultural values of their professions. The emphasis on acute work is the setting in which medicine is most likely to dominate, so it is where there is most likely to be variants in any transition from a subordinate nursing role to a complementary interprofessional relationship.

The boundary between occupations is often a site of tension and change as a result of technical developments in the labour process and wider social transformations. That doctors and nurses have to form a team to provide adequately for their patients is widely accepted, and an acceptance that the team benefits from leadership is equally uncontentious, but the question of who provides that leadership can be vigorously contested.

Interprofessional working

Medicine and nursing are ostensibly distinguished by the different functions they perform within health care. The sphere of the doctor is seen as being to diagnose and treat, while that of the nurse is to care. Leaving aside for the moment the question of whether it is feasible to distinguish clearly between 'care' and 'treatment', the relationship between these two spheres of action contains two competing principles. In one there is a hierarchy in which the nurse is simply the doctor's 'handmaid', and in the other medicine and nursing are complementary professions. Nursing staff who are willing to accept a subordinate role will accept medical leadership, and are unlikely to assert the importance of patient care where this does not fit a ward agenda dominated by the priorities of senior doctors. Where nurses are determined to give priority to patient care they will not accept medical control of the nursing agenda. Many nurses are resistant to the role of doctor's handmaiden in modern hospitals. How this relationship between the professions is affected by the gendering of the professions, which itself is changing as more women become doctors and more senior nurses men, is a further issue.

Both medicine and nursing aspire to the highest standards of professionalism. However, this has different meanings both within the two professions and to sociologists. The process by which occupations seek to professionalise has been a dominant theme in the analysis of professions, addressing the negotiation and struggles over the creation and maintenance of boundaries with other occupations and professions.

There have been varying models of cooperation between medicine and nursing. Medical consultants have always had legal and organisational responsibility for patient care. From the beginning of the NHS they have been involved in managing hospitals. Generally, before the 1960s, a typical pattern was of fairly static ward nursing teams of qualified nursing staff dominated by a ward sister who deferred to the consultant on all substantive issues of patient care management. In 1968 the Salmon Committee recommended substantial change to what they perceived as an anachronistic pattern. The nursing profession was remodelled to conform to a line management structure with carefully defined areas of nursing responsibility for each grade. Gradually medical involvement in nurse training diminished or disappeared and consultant doctors ceased to be involved in nursing appointments. The authority of nurse managers was vigorously contested at times by medical staff.

The introduction of general management in 1985 reduced the status of senior nursing staff, and destroyed a career structure that had been exclusively available to nurses, but on the wards clinical nurse managers remained in post, so that medical–nursing relationships were not substantially affected. Concurrently, and in various locations in many countries, nursing developed systems for organising a more personal form of patient care that recognised the need of an ill person to have individual care. 'Primary nursing' has many of the attributes extolled by new wave managers; there is autonomy for the primary nurse, responsiveness to patient requirements, and a potential for excellence. Leadership is from the nursing profession. Primary nursing has developed independently of medical involvement. Many nurses now perceive themselves as responsible for providing care as distinct from treatment, and as having their own body of research-based expertise to draw on to determine optimum patterns of care provision. Emphasis is on holistic care of the entire person and providing an advocacy for the patient as a vulnerable person within hospitals.

The changes in the boundary between medicine and nursing with the development of new medical technology and the reorganisation of health work are crucial for understanding the interprofessional relations of doctors and nurses. With the continuing attempts to reduce the hours of junior doctors (NHS Management Executive, 1991), increasing interest in shifting some tasks to nurses, and the renewed professionalisation project of nurses seeking to upskill their occupation (UKCC, 1986), the negotiation of the complex boundary between the tasks of medicine and nursing is a matter of pressing policy concern.

Our study shows that the two professions have a complicated relationship which is mediated by a number of principles involving both difference and complementarity, on the one hand, and hierarchy and subordination, on the other. In investigating the nature of the boundary between doctors and nurses we discovered new complexities which are not a matter of simple hierarchy. There are different notions of professionalism at stake stemming from the different circumstances of doctors and nurses and which in turn give rise to complex forms of interaction. The increasingly fragmented time and space geography of hospitals causes problems for cooperation between the professions yet this fragmentation is exacerbated by the search for efficiency and increased throughput of patients. Rival principles of efficiency compete – either sub-divide, monitor and regulate or be flexible, holistic and trust – paralleling the debate on Fordism and post-Fordism.

The substantive study at the heart of this book has as its focus the health service and the working relationships of the two key groups of health workers: doctors and nurses. We ask about the pressures on its key workers in the context of a health service undergoing significant change. Health workers are an increasingly significant section of the workforce, and part of the growing service sector. We focus on the relations of two adjacent occupations, on the nature of the boundary between them, and how it is being negotiated. When are these workers allies and when adversaries? These are traditionally gendered occupations, but they are undergoing significant changes as women enter medicine and, to some extent, men enter nursing. What difference, if any, does gender make to the relations of these occupations? And what can this contribute to our understanding of contemporary gender relations?

The focus of the empirical work is firmly based on the day-to-day work of hospital doctors and nurses. Just as the imperative of new wave management and post-Fordist conceptualisation is on the workers at the cutting edge of production, so for our focus we concentrate on two groups of professional staff who are directly involved in delivering care and treatment. If the constant changes that are made to health service organisation do not make the work of these two groups more effective, then the value of change has to be questioned. If leadership is as pivotal to corporate activity as is claimed, then the factors associated with leadership, and the potential for effective leadership in multi-professional teams needs to be better understood. This requires a clear understanding of how professional boundaries can serve patient interests, and the implications of their being dismantled or by-passed.

The boundary between medicine and nursing is one of the best places to investigate interprofessional relations. This is the point where pressures for change and differences of view can be most easily seen. Conflict at this point is an indicator of these pressures, and of the differences between the professions. Conflict is often seen as a problem to be eradicated if at all possible, and some forms of conflict are indeed simply negative and wearing to the protagonists, but in the case of interprofessional relations conflict is not always and necessarily a bad thing. The patient gains the benefit of a robust discussion of his or her interests from more than one viewpoint. In our study we use conflict at the boundary of the two professions as an indicator of differences of view and of pressures for change.

The research study

The book draws upon several sources of data, including interviews with 262 doctors and nurses, printed sources, interviews with key informants and secondary data. The interview study proceeded at a number of levels. The empirical focus was to collect the data necessary to map the patterns of conflict and cooperation between doctors and nurses in a wide range of contexts. Our middle range interest was in the contrasting range of working practices in a changing NHS. How were the specifics of the interprofessional relations in health to be understood? At a further level we were interested in the processes of negotiation of occupational boundaries.

The research project was focused around in-depth interviews with a varied sample of 127 doctors and 135 nurses in 1990–91. The response rate was just over 90 per cent, with only 28 of the 290 initially selected respondents being unable or unwilling to be interviewed. Among the doctors 97 were male and 30 were female and among the nurses 19 were male and 116 were female. The doctors and nurses were distributed through the range of grades. Among the doctors there were 30 consultants, 11 senior registrars, 28 registrars, 35 senior house officers and 23 house officers. Among the nurses there were 55 sisters/charge nurses and 80 staff nurses.

In order to be able to ask about the significance of different working contexts these were spread through five hospitals and seven medical specialties. The five hospitals are called in the text City, College, County, Central and Greenfield. They include two teaching hospitals and three non-teaching hospitals. Two were in Scotland, one in London and two in other parts of England. All names are imaginary and do not relate to any hospital thus named. The freedom with which respondents gave information was impressive and their anonymity has been carefully protected. The medical specialties were: medicine 64 interviews; surgery 51; ENT 20; psychiatry 30; care of the elderly 37; ICU 36; paediatrics 15; theatre and A&E 9 (surgeons were counted as part of the surgical sample, not that of theatre). The specialties were located in a range of hospitals, but it was not possible to find each specialty in every institution (see Appendix).

The research included a variety of other groups of interest. One was a group of people who had been both doctors and nurses themselves. Unit general managers at our hospitals were another. Seventeen interviews were conducted with nursing officers/nurse managers. Professional bodies of doctors and nurses were also contacted. A discussion group of medical and nursing students was held by a trained facilitator. Various other constituencies were approached at different stages of the research, such as the Schools of Nursing and Medical Schools. A certain amount of observation of the working practices was possible on visits to hospitals.

The structure of the book

Chapter 2 explores the nature of professional boundaries in NHS hospitals. We show that a division between care and treatment is an inadequate base on which to distinguish between professions. We will argue that while some aspects of the traditional theories of professions are reinforced (both doctors and nurses are committed to professionalism and professional projects and there are a few issues of conflict at the task boundary) others need reassessment (for instance, less conflict over increasing nurse skill than is predicted). We suggest that the professionalisation strategy of nurses is advancing, but that the profession itself, by emphasising rule-bound behaviour, limits the autonomy of nurses.

Chapter 3 provides a theoretical context to understand the data on professional boundaries. We examine the literature on the sociology of professions and segmented and segregated labour markets. The developments in the medical and nursing professions are examined in this context.

A significant set of these issues relates to the increasingly fragmented time–space geography of modern hospitals which is exacerbated by the search for efficiencies in an environment of fierce cost containment. Chapter 4 addresses these areas of tension along the boundary between doctors and nurses which are not captured by the traditional notions of interprofessional competition. We note the evidence that hospitals are organised along Fordist principles in order to maximise productivity, with some loss of quality in the levels of care that can be given. We describe contrasts between hospitals, and indicate possible links with both different funding patterns and qualities of leadership. We summarise the factors likely to have positive and negative impacts on interprofessional team working.

Chapter 5 considers the management of professional workers in contemporary NHS hospitals. We consider the implications of the different modes of organisation of medicine and nursing on their negotiation of working practices especially at the boundary and its possible role in conflicts. We consider the tensions between new and old forms of management and its relation to and implications for professional modes of governance.

Finally, Chapter 6 asks whether the changing nature of interprofessional relations can be understood in terms of a move towards a post-Fordist mode of regulation. We argue for the relevance of the tensions between Fordist and post-Fordist logics of organisation to the practice of, not only medicine and nursing, but wider social relations.

2

Professional Boundaries

A central characteristic of post-Fordism is that large hierarchical organisations are replaced by small semi-autonomous units. New wave management is an organisational expression of the same trend. The changes to the NHS that were outlined in *Working for Patients* (Department of Health, 1989a) involved devolution of authority and ownership to smaller units – NHS Trusts and GP budget holders – in a way that is consistent with post-Fordist principles. The effect of NHS change on other values, are not discussed in this chapter.

Devolution to independent organisations is only one aspect of new wave management. The crucial element is devolution of responsibility down to the staff who are 'close to the customer', and in health care this means the staff who are caring for patients. The development of GP budget holding appears to fit within 'new wave' principles, but the creation of Trusts is a process of devolving authority to an institution, and does not in itself guarantee that the staff who are 'close to the customer' will gain greater control over decision making. Individual Trusts would have to be studied to see how far the process of internal devolution has been implemented.

There are other aspects of NHS change that indicate a loss of autonomy by clinical staff rather than a gain, particularly because of the need to operate within the tightly defined financial limits of service contracts. There is nothing new in having limits on health service spending, and some of the critical comments on Trust hospital finance applied equally to health authorities before 1991, but the need for each Trust to win its own contracts in order to secure its own future has imposed a greater discipline on financial management, and inevitably this limits clinical autonomy. Furthermore, Trusts require a strengthened management function, building on the general management principles introduced in 1985. So a post-Fordist process of devolving authority to semi-autonomous Trusts is proceeding alongside a strengthened management process that may operate in ways more akin to Taylorism or Fordism. That the resulting impact is somewhat confused is not surprising.

Nevertheless, the process of devolving authority within hospitals has continued with the formation of clinical directorates, i.e. groupings of similar specialties with their own budgets. It is an indication that authority is moving downward, closer to the ward and clinics where patients are treated. The practicalities of achieving good-quality service provision within defined budgets is the dominant theme, and this requires collaboration between groups of separately organised professionals and non-professional staff. If decision making is to be devolved downwards – in the interests of both patients and workers – then a central issue is how professions which are independently structured can form effective interprofessional teams.

For some professions – education is an example – interprofessional relations is not a significant issue. In education, service provision is dominated by a single profession, albeit one with several sub-groups. By contrast, providing a health care service requires several professions to work closely and continuously together, not just at an occasional interprofessional liaison committee, but day-by-day in clinics, surgeries and hospitals. Devolving authority downwards increases the need to form effective interprofessional teams because it is at the 'team' level that decisions have to be made. At the same time, bringing some decision making to a team level potentially reduces the influence of professions who operate through hierarchical structures. So devolving decision making is a process with particular implications for the health professions.

Quite apart from structural changes, there are other immediate and practical issues that are also concurrently forcing attention onto the nature of health service collaboration. The policy of reducing junior doctors' hours by transferring some tasks from junior doctors to other staff is particularly relevant. The transfer of services from long-stay hospitals to families, or community-based residential care, brings into sharper focus the balance of authority between the professions. Attempting to evaluate the outcome of treatment focuses attention on the contribution of several professions and the extent to which their work is interdependent.

In this book we are examining empirical data only from hospitals, and concentrating only on medical and nursing interaction. The question of how best to organise interprofessional health care teams is not restricted to hospital wards but, nevertheless, it remains the case that the overwhelming majority of health professionals begin their careers in hospital, and absorb ideas of appropriate professional relations from working patterns developed in hospital. The variety of practice that exists in hospitals also allows for a greater understanding of how patterns of collaboration develop, though at the same time the complexity of hospital organisation highlights the way that locally specific factors affect the nature of professional working relations. The interdependent nature of medical and nursing work, their central role in health care delivery, and their varied historical patterns of professionalisation, make the inter-professional relations of these two groups particularly significant.

How in practice do the two professions of medicine and nursing work together? Is nursing subservient to medicine, or are both professions dependent on each other, embracing a symbiotic and complementary relationship? Does medicine determine where the boundary is between the two professions, and set limits to the skill and influence of nursing so as to ensure its own dominance? Or has nursing claimed effective control over an area of expertise from which doctors are excluded? The wider context of the historical construction of these gendered professions as differently positioned in relation to sources of social power is discussed in the next chapter.

For some aspects of clinical activity these current substantive questions can be answered easily. Within hospitals, medicine determines many significant decisions. Doctors, particularly consultants, decide who will be admitted to hospital and when patients can be discharged. They make the diagnosis and they control treatment decisions. Nurses work within these parameters in deciding the appropriate care pattern for particular patients. So while there are many aspects of hospital nursing that are determined wholly by nurses, there are other aspects of the care that nurses give to patients, for example, the administration of drugs and the prep-aration of patients for surgery, which are determined by medical decisions. Figure 2.1a illustrates this.

An alternative view is that nursing is an entirely separate profession, one that has a stronger relationship with medical

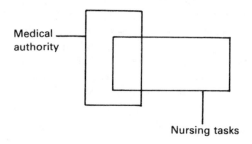

Figure 2.1a *Medical control of nursing tasks*

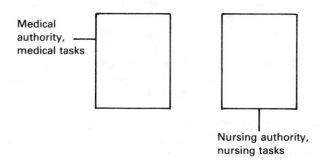

Medical
authority,
medical tasks

Nursing authority,
nursing tasks

Figure 2.1b   *Separate spheres of influence of medicine and nursing*

colleagues than with other health service professionals. The spheres of influence are seen as entirely separate (Figure 2.1b). A third concept places nursing within a hierarchical system controlled by consultants (Figure 2.1c). This is how one consultant described the ward sister's role:

> *Consultant*:   A ward sister . . . runs the place in [the doctor's] absence and she is like the sergeant-major who then gives the next tier, like the nurses, the orders of what needs to be done. So if you clash with the sister, that's a problem, there's a complete obstruction in the middle between the commander and the troops.

This description fails to give any notion of the large area of nursing practice unconnected with medical decision making, and conveys a sense of obedient submission that has largely disappeared from UK nursing. A doctor who expects this pattern would be bound to clash with a nursing colleague committed to the concept of nursing as an

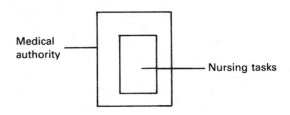

Medical
authority

Nursing tasks

Figure 2.1c   *Nursing wholly within consultants' control*

entirely separate profession, and is also likely to define the boundary between medicine and nursing in ways that are unacceptable even to nurses who recognise some measure of medical influence over their work.

The exact nature of medical–nursing interaction varies to some extent between specialties, but wherever the boundary lies, there are a series of questions that need to be asked. Do nurses accept medical control over admission, diagnosis, treatment and discharge? Is the boundary between medicine and nursing clearly defined and accepted, or fuzzy and contested? Is it imposed through a professional hierarchy, or can it normally be negotiated by the ward-based staff who provide patient care? Most important of all, do the existing patterns best serve the needs of patients? Can professionals from different groups manage the boundaries between themselves in ways that give primacy to patient interests? When the boundaries of medicine and nursing are contested, is the patient called into the argument only to give an alibi for professional self-interest, or is patient well-being an effective arbiter in interprofessional disputes?

In the research project outlined in Chapter 1, we asked doctors and nurses about the boundaries between their areas of responsibility; their perception of interprofessional teamwork; and the issues that had recently caused conflict between them. These are professionals whose stated priority is the care of the patient, but who sometimes think the best interest of the patient is served in different ways. We are emphasising the areas of disagreement not because we want to suggest that these are disrupting the care of the patient to a dangerous extent, although there is clearly room for improvement on a number of issues, but because this provides the best way of understanding the negotiation of the changing division of labour between health professionals.

Over 400 incidents of recent nurse–doctor conflict were recorded. Analysis of them showed that there were 15 types of conflict, and that these related to three major categories. Details are shown in Table 2.1. This chapter focuses on the first category, the conflict situations that relate to divisions and boundaries of professional authority and responsibility, and those that give some indication of the extent to which the professions 'put patients first' in the management of clinical work. The second category, which we have referred to as 'time–space geography under pressure', is discussed in Chapter 4. It is here that the impact of pressure on NHS services becomes apparent. The influence of professional culture, personality and attitude (the third category) is evident throughout the text, there is no one chapter relating specifically to this category.

Table 2.1 *Conflict-related issues reported by doctors and nurses*

	Number of responses indicating conflict or anger		
	Doctor	Nurse	Total
Professional boundaries in question	107	114	221
Different opinions regarding treatment	22	27	49
Different task priorities	27	18	45
Controlling bad practice	20	19	39
Intervention in the care of dying patients	9	14	23
Won't listen; won't acknowledge colleague's expertise	8	11	19
Doctor–nurse manager conflict	17	1	18
Lack of respect/courtesy to patients	2	13	15
Doctor–doctor conflict affecting treatment/care	2	11	13
Time–space geography under pressure	64	82	146
Bleep	20	24	44
Low staffing cover/tiredness/stress	21	13	34
Bed allocation, admission, discharge	5	22	27
Communication failure	10	15	25
Theatre lists over time	8	8	16
Individual and other factors	22	34	56
Personality/attitude to colleagues	12	26	38
Comments not allocated	10	8	18
Total			423

These accounts of conflict are used to examine three questions in this chapter. First, in section A: Contested Authority we attempt to clarify the nature of the hierarchical relationship between the two professions. We do this by examining accounts of different opinions about treatments; different task priorities; doctor-nurse manager conflicts; and intra-medical conflicts. Secondly, in many of the conversations with nursing and medical staff the impression was conveyed that there was a clear distinction between 'treatment' and 'care', with doctors controlling treatment, while nursing staff managed care. This is examined in section B: Care or Treatment, using examples of treatment disputes linked to the care-treatment boundary issue. Wound management, intensive care nursing, and the care of dying patients are significant areas. In section C: Patients First? we are concerned to see if patients' interests act as an arbiter in patterns of inter-professional conflict, and how disputes over issues of respect and courtesy to patients are managed.

A: CONTESTED AUTHORITY

Medicine has already been described as having a dominant position in hospitals by having authority over admissions, treatment decisions and discharge of patients, but this does not give doctors control over the work of other health professions. So how is authority negotiated?

(i) Control of treatment

When doctors and nurses were asked to describe the difference between medical and nursing responsibilities a frequent response was to say that treatment was a medical concern, or that doctors provided treatment, and nursing staff managed the care of patients. Given the large number of conflicts generated by different opinions over treatment these statements need to be re-assessed.

We found that many of the conflicts over treatment related to the balance of authority between newly qualified doctors and experienced nurses. Professional boundaries, as well as the extent of authority, are least well defined when patients are being seen by a very junior doctor.

> *SHO*:   When I qualified I had this sort of rosy idea that the doctors would prescribe and nurses would administer . . . which is not the case! . . . [nurses] put a lot of pressure on you if they feel the patient should have one drug and you feel that another is more appropriate.

> *Staff nurse*:   We have just had the junior doctors start . . . straight out of university, and they are like babies put out in this wide world . . . Drugs, they don't know what drugs are normally used . . . for instance if a patient's got cardiac pain you know automatically what is given . . . Now they don't know that, and they have their formulary and they are kind of flicking through the pages, while meanwhile the man is gasping . . . and you have got to try and, not tell them, but nicely advise that, perhaps, you know, they could use this particular drug . . . but . . . you have got to be very diplomatic, depending again on the doctor. You are frightened to go over the mark.

We found that arguments over diagnosis were characteristically arguments over a provisional diagnosis, later confirmed or rejected by the consultant or senior registrar. Almost all doctors below the level of consultant are in 'training' posts. In challenging junior doctors' decisions, nurses are taking the training designation of the junior doctor at face value. Their challenge is justified by their duty to query instructions that they think are not in the patient's interest, so such challenges could, theoretically, be equally made to the consultant, but in practice this is rare. The pattern appears to be that nursing staff accept the authority of a consultant, and of doctors in the more senior grades of training posts, but experienced nurses challenge the decisions of younger doctors, or doctors whose decisions are out of line with normal ward practice. Senior medical staff usually support them.

A frequent criticism from nurses is that doctors simply will not listen to what they have to say about a patient. 'They hear, but they won't listen.' Doctors find it equally irritating that nurses will close off discussion of a patient's condition, but then refuse to accept their decision. Both professions nevertheless insist that an effective exchange of information is vital if patients are to be cared for adequately.

> *Senior registrar*:   There are nurses down there that have been at the job for 20 years, and a lot of them are better at pattern recognition for ECGs [electrocardiograph, to record the electrical discharges produced by heart tissue] and things like that than I am. I think that the circumstances under which their opinions are not listened to are with very junior anaesthetists who have got some sort of attitude into their head that they know more about intensive care than the nursing staff do, which when they start is completely wrong, and that is definitely a source of conflict here.

There were considerable cultural and national variations in the extent to which nurses contested doctors' decisions. Expressions of deference were observed more frequently in Scotland. Mackay (1993) discusses aspects of our research findings that relate to differences in professional cultures in England and Scotland. Most UK hospitals have some staff who have trained outside the UK. Their expectations of interprofessional relations vary with dominant UK patterns. The range of cultural attitudes within the UK is also considerable.

In the five hospitals where interviews were conducted, we met nursing staff who resented the attitude of German-trained medical staff, and their expectation that they would always be accompanied and assisted by nursing staff when attending to patients; an Indian doctor who was delighted that nursing staff managed the dressings on a surgical ward without medical staff involvement; a South African doctor who was impressed by the extent to which nursing staff in the UK familiarised themselves with the details of their patients' home circumstances; several non-UK trained doctors who were surprised by what they perceived to be over-tight restrictions on what nursing staff were allowed to monitor or manage; three nurses who noted greater formality in medical attitudes in the UK than they were used to in the USA and Australia. Comments were also made indicating that cultural attitudes which ascribed an inferior status to women caused some interprofessional friction, and differences between teaching and district general hospitals, and the rapidity of social change in the UK were also noted. The variations expressed indicate the necessity of caution in making global statements. The use of the term 'girls' to refer to nurses is common, together with the Scottish 'girlies'. These extracts give some idea of the range of attitudes.

> *Registrar*:   Here [nurses] are definitely better qualified and trained and their outlook is different. In India nurses are very much subordinate, there is a different hierarchical system there. They don't . . . put their point forward because they know that doctors would not listen to them. They just follow their [doctors'] instructions, but here everyone speaks their own mind and they do not hesitate to speak up and say something. I really admire them for that. Indian doctors find it difficult to understand the system. Fresh from India it takes some time to find out how it all works.

> *Staff nurse*:   In Australia . . . [nurses] follow a lot closer on the heels of America. So they are a lot more up to date in what they are doing and they are a lot more forward looking than what I have seen here. There's a lot more team spirit involved in all aspects of nursing and doctoring out there.

> *Staff nurse*:   When I started here it was very formal and it reflected back on the doctors. In London it was always first-name terms . . . here it was 'staff nurse' and 'sister' and sister stood up when the doctors came in. Only sister sat down and staff nurses stood. We were not really working as a team when I started here.
> [So what caused it to change?]
> Oh, one of the senior sisters left.

> *Consultant*:   I noticed the girls down here to be particularly interested in their jobs. It is very common for a student nurse to just come straight up and ask what's wrong or why are you doing this or argue with your management of a patient as a perfect matter of course. It would be much more of a hierarchical approach in a teaching hospital . . . I don't mind either way, but it is much more interesting to be questioned . . . In the teaching hospitals there is a lot of questioning of roles and this sort of thing, but here the doctors tend to agree with me and it's the girls that take over the role of the questioned!

There were frequent conflicts over who was actually responsible for carrying out particular treatments. Two examples are intravenous drug and fluid administration and the wider issue of responsibility for drugs.

Intravenous drug and fluid administration The management of intravenous drugs (IVs) was frequently mentioned as being a 'boundary' area between the responsibilities of doctors and nurses. Junior doctors were sometimes intense in their criticism of current practice of allocation of responsibilities, which they largely ascribed to the influence of nurse managers. Ironically, and in contrast to the intensity with which this issue was discussed, there were few reported incidents of conflict, largely because medical staff knew that practice was regulated by policies outside the control of the nurses that they met on the wards. Box 2.1 gives a description of the technique and background of the procedure of IV fluid and drug administration for readers unfamiliar with the practice.

The question of whether doctors or nurses should give IV drugs draws on several issues, particularly that of whether a particular task is sufficiently complex and interventionist to warrant being a doctor's task as it was originally, or now simple and routine enough to become a nurse's job. However, there are issues other than simplicity at stake, including nurse management policies, hospital board policies and consideration of patient needs. Nurses who have undertaken post-qualifying certification courses that give them an 'extended role' are authorised to do much of this IV work.

> *House officer*: A lot of hospital nurses can do IV drugs as long as they have done the recommended course . . . this health board won't allow any nurses to do these courses . . . if I have got a lot of things to do, giving IV antibiotics is way down on the list, and it means that IVs that should be given at 8 o'clock are sometimes given at 10 o'clock, because it is simply the least urgent.

> *Registrar*: That has always annoyed me, the fact that nurses aren't allowed to do things that a monkey could do . . . it is becoming worse . . . the crazy thing [is] even if you have got qualifications to do coronary care where you are allowed to give intravenous drugs, once you come out of coronary care you are not allowed to do it . . . it is so stupid.

The question as to whether doctors or nurses should do IVs is a matter of general discussion in the two professions. For instance, the Standing Committee on Postgraduate Medical Education (SCOPME) sees the administration of intravenous drugs as one of three tasks which should be transferred from junior doctors to nurses (SCOPME, 1991).

In our study the administration of IVs was raised as an issue of contention in some units, while in others it was never mentioned. Conflict was most evident in those hospitals where different wards and specialties had markedly different policies. So in one hospital

Intravenous (IV) fluid and drug administration

IVs are the administration of fluids or the injection of drugs directly into the vein, that is, intravenously. This form of drug administration is used because it is the most rapid way of causing drugs to enter and act on the body. A further advantage of this procedure is that it by-passes the digestive tract which could alter the nature of the drugs and is available when patients are unable to take drugs orally. There is an increasing use of IVs as a route for drug administration. Various drugs can be administered intravenously including pain-killers, antibiotics and other drugs which correct imbalances in body functions. IV fluids, such as saline and glucose, can be given to those patients who cannot drink or are unable to take in fluids at the necessary rate. (For instance, burns patients lose a lot of body fluid which needs to be constantly replenished.)

There are a number of complexities inherent in the procedure which can cause problems, such as the risk of blood clotting, the need to regulate the drip flow carefully, the risk of infection (sepsis), the possibility of the drip running through with the risk of air entering the body (potentially fatal), and that of a sudden negative reaction to the drug which is entering the body very rapidly.

The procedure is to insert a needle into a vein. If IV fluids are required or if IV drugs need to be administered on several occasions, a narrow tube, a cannula, is left in the vein so that there is not the need to 'cut down' into the vein on each occasion. Normally the vein would be kept open by being attached to a saline drip. There are several further technical features, such as a heparin lock, to prevent blood clotting at the point of entry. A further development has been the use of central venous lines. These are long cannulas, usually inserted into a neck vein and then through to a large vein near the heart. It is possible to provide all the daily nutrients required through a central line. In order to stop these long cannulas from blocking, it is essential to flush them with a saline solution in between giving more dense liquids.

These procedures have developed rapidly over the past 20 years. The earliest procedure was the one-off injection of drugs into veins. The development of semi-permanent drips was a significant shift in medical practice made possible by a number of technical developments (such as special tubing to which blood did not stick, the heparin lock to prevent blood clotting, and the increase in the number of drugs available which can be used in this way). Central venous lines are a further development. The change in technology with the use of fixed cannulas means that the procedure is more routine, simpler and safer than before, presenting fewer possibilities for complications. IV drug administration is now considered routine work.

Historically the doctor has given all IV injections and put up the IV drip. While nurses gave injections into muscles or into the skin, they did not do so into veins. The giving of drugs so rapidly has potential life-threatening consequences and this, together with the complexity of the early procedures, were reasons for the task being considered a medical rather than nursing one. Nurses changed the bottles and bags holding the fluids which are being fed into the veins, and managed the drips the doctor had set up.

where IV drugs were managed by doctors in all the wards except the Intensive Care Unit there was little conflict. On wards where there were sufficient nurses with extended role qualifications to manage this work there was also little conflict. It was when a particular ward or department did not train sufficient extended role nurses to do the work, while other wards did, that IV drug administration led to nurse–doctor conflict.

The majority of doctors were in favour of nurses doing IVs. Of the 95 doctors in our study who addressed this issue, 74 (78 per cent) said that nurses should do so. By contrast, less than half the nurses were in favour, 41 (48 per cent) of the 85 who addressed the issue thought that this should be a nurse's job, although in practice 73 per cent presently give or are prepared to give them. Not only did the views of the doctors and nurses over who should do the task diverge, but there were divisions within each profession. Among doctors it tended to be the more senior who did not approve of nurses doing IV drugs (not the junior doctors whose task it might be).

There are variations between different units in a hospital, between different hospitals, and between different health authorities (England and Wales) and health boards (Scotland). Some health authorities/boards have retreated from enlarging this programme as a result of one instance of difficulty with a nurse administering the drug. One nurse in our study was halfway through her extended role training when this was stopped after there was an incident to which the health authority reacted by restricting the policy of training nurses in this way.

The issues involved in these divisions of opinion do not include the level of technical competence of the nurses, since almost everyone agrees that a nurse could do it (if given the available training). The technical ability needed to do the task itself is quite simple, but an awareness of all the potential complications and dangers make it a task which is not handed to a newly qualified nurse.

In interview, nurses gave two main reasons for resenting and opposing the transfer of responsibility for the management of IV drugs from doctors to nurses. One was a matter of containing the size of the workload of nurses, and this in turn was linked to the question of nurse staffing levels. On many wards, probably most wards, nurses felt themselves to be understaffed and not able to provide the level of nursing care that they wished to give. Taking over responsibility for IV drugs would mean taking on a time-consuming task when there was an overwhelming conviction that no extra qualified nursing staff would be provided. To create time to give IV drugs, qualified nurses may have to hand over to non-qualified staff duties that nurses considered to be extremely important for patient care, but non-nursing managers treated as less important. Some nurses felt that their proper job was to relate to patients as people and have time to talk to them, to deal with their concerns, make sure of their comfort, speak to their relatives and not merely to carry out technical procedures. These areas were being squeezed out by the pressures of work. So for some nurses, though not all, the central concern was to protect the agenda of nursing, so that nursing could develop as a distinctive, caring and holistic response to patients' needs. For such nurses, IV drug administration had to be firmly placed as a task that nurses may help with, but which remained, ultimately, a medical task.

> *Ward sister*: There isn't always a nurse who can do it . . . like on the ward next door to us . . . If we're busy one of the doctors will have to do it. It's their responsibility to make sure that the drugs are given. If we can't do it, then they have to . . . [the doctor] might be angry but that's his problem. I'm sorry for that but I'm not going to feel guilty about it . . . you've got to understand that the nurses aren't always going to be there to see to it, you know, they [the doctors] need to be aware of what is actually in their responsibility, and one of them is the administration of drugs, to see that the drugs are given.

Some nurses and doctors agreed that it was better for patients if nurses gave IV drugs because then they would be given on time. More nurses than doctors mentioned the benefits to patients. These are significant because blood levels of drugs must be consistently maintained and this requires prompt administration when the drug is due, commonly every six hours. So referring the debate back to what was in the patient's interest provided a mutual basis for agreement, though qualified by a nursing concern over adequate staffing, and the need to give priority to nursing duties. Apart from the benefit to patients, there were seen to be advantages for nurses, in that it was less stressful to get on with the task than to wait for the doctor.

The risk of insurance claims was raised by some respondents as a reason for nurses not undertaking IVs. Historically, hospitals have been responsible for medical insurance claims arising out of nurses' actions. Until recently, it was not responsible for claims of negligence against doctors. Some of our medical respondents felt that the lack of eagerness to see that there were adequate numbers of extended role nurses related to the hospital authorities' concerns about insurance costs. However, this opinion was roundly rejected by unit managers who said that the issues were not related at all. Current changes in the 'extended role' policy are discussed below.

In some ways the trajectory of the development of the division of labour over IVs is similar to that of other procedures, such as those of muscular injections. A newly introduced procedure is likely to be performed by a doctor, but as it is refined and simplified with technical advances and becomes routine there is pressure for it to be handed over to nurses, or to other paramedical occupations.

Prescribing and administering drugs   Doctors prescribe drugs and nurses administer them (except for some IV drugs). Nurses are required by their professional code of practice to work in a collaborative and cooperative manner with other professions involved in health care, and to ensure that nothing they do is detrimental to the safety of patients. They must decline to carry out tasks that they think are detrimental to the safety of patients. These dual obligations to collaborate, and at the same time to decline to undertake duties that they are not certain are safe, gives rise to particular tensions over the administration of drugs. Irritation and conflict is most common in connection with prescribing at night.

For junior doctors a particular cause of irritation concerns prescriptions for mild analgesics. When a patient has woken up in some pain, and needs some paracetamol – a mild pain-killer for sale in most supermarkets outside hospital – the nurse has to have a doctor's authorisation. Usually the situation will have been fore-seen, and the doctor will have written up the drug 'p.r.n.' – as needed. If it has not been anticipated that the patient would be in pain, and there is no prescription, the nurse needs to inform the doctor, and get a prescription. In the middle of the night this involves bleeping the doctor, who may be snatching a few hours of sleep in a weekend 'on-call' duty. It is infuriating to junior medical staff. (We came to realise that the commercial name for paraceta-mol has become so much of a symbol of nursing attitudes that it is sufficient in itself to generate impassioned outbursts from house officers.) For an exhausted house officer, having to be woken by an experienced nurse to authorise mild analgesics is caution carried to extreme. While some nurses bend the rules, and some doctors encourage them to do so, others feel that the only safe option is to stick with the formal procedure. Listening to junior doctors and staff nurses discussing this issue is a reminder of the strength of cultural differences between the professions.

> *Staff nurse*:   I never give [analgesics] without the doctor's information. I'd ring him up, and we're allowed to take verbal messages and sign for it, and then the doctors will have to sign it later . . . but I wouldn't just give it, because you never know . . . I'm not prepared to take responsibility for just giving somebody paracetamol, I know they can

> go out and they can buy it, . . . but you have to work within the guide-line. I'm really thinking . . . I suppose when you do your extended roles, when you're working you're thinking I don't want to lose my registration, you know, so you have to work within the guide-line.

This staff nurse mentioned that she was allowed to take 'verbals'. Being able to give a verbal means that the doctor can, over the phone, tell the nurse that a patient can have a particular drug, and does not have actually to go to the ward to write down the prescription personally. Usually the message has to be received by two nurses as a means of confirming the dose and preventing error. Formal rules are variably implemented, so in a hospital that forbids verbals, junior doctors may find that on one ward they are required to go to the ward at 3.00 am to order a particular drug, while on an adjacent ward a nurse will allow the prescription to be given over the phone, though strictly she should not do so.

> *Senior house officer*: They always take a verbal here, but some places you know they won't even take a verbal, you would have to physically go and sign for it, yes honest to God . . . it was atrocious. Really, at X hospital, they weren't allowed to take verbals over the phone, and the sister or the charge nurse would be going over the phone (whispering) 'Well, if you sign for it as soon as you come' but they weren't supposed to.

For many junior doctors, a nurse who conforms to a rule that forbids verbals is someone who won't accept professional responsibility, while for some nurses refusing to accept the authority of rules is equally clear evidence of unprofessional behaviour. Nurses and doctors will bend the rules if they know each other well enough to trust each other's judgement, and if they are confident enough of their own position. As will be discussed in Chapter 4, whether or not this is possible depends partly on whether there are stable teams of permanent staff.

(ii) Task priorities

Both doctors and nurses report anger and conflict situations over tasks that are not carried out by the other profession. This is the second largest type of conflict and is partly linked to the question of having authority to decide on priorities, but relates also to the different 'geography' of medical and nursing work in hospital. If medicine and nursing are hierarchical in their relationship, then the doctor can decide on priorities. If not, how are task priorities to be decided, particularly when the work load of nurses is located on a particular ward, while doctors work over several wards, and departments?

Doctors will give priority to tasks either on the basis of immediate medical needs over several wards, or as determined by their consultants' timetables. The priorities of ward nursing staff are set primarily by the needs of the patients on their ward, adjusted to allow for other priorities such as the handover of information to the next shift of nurses, seeing relatives, or accompanying the consultant on a ward round. A registrar described the process of establishing his priorities as 'a war of attrition' with nursing staff. Ward nursing staff do not have the right to impose their priorities on junior doctors, and doctors cannot enforce a request that something is done promptly. When a patient is seriously ill the priorities for both groups of staff will be the same, and the treatment programme confirmed by a consultant after a ward round also establishes some priorities, but for much of the time both groups of staff have different priorities that are established by the nature of their professional responsibilities.

Handmaidens? A particular aspect of 'different task priorities' concerns tidying up after treatment procedures have been carried out. The question of whether a nurse should tidy up after a doctor was not spontaneously raised in most interviews, and was included as a specific question only after early interviews had shown it was a contentious issue. The question of tidying up is one of the clearest indicators of whether there is a hierarchical relationship between the professions or not. The underlying issue is whether nurses should be treated as doctors' 'handmaidens'. Nurses see themselves as having been regarded in this way in the past and most are determined to claim their position as independent professionals. Where nurses are strongly committed to this view they increasingly insist on doctors tidying up after themselves.

The question of tidying up is both trivial and important simultaneously.

> *Sister*: Untidiness is a mammoth problem. It is *really* irritating, and we tell them every day of the week we are not here to clear up after you . . . they just leave the place an *absolute* tip. If they use something they leave it where they last used it, they wouldn't dream of putting it away . . . and it is infuriating.

Many respondents commented that it was such a routine issue that they had not thought to raise it, but subsequent to including it in our interview schedule, 79 per cent of doctors and 82 per cent of nurses reported that it caused difficulties. Our question was: 'There are specific things that have been reported to us as often causing conflict. One of them is tidying up and who is responsible for tidying up. Does this cause difficulties for you?' This usually met with a laugh from the interviewee, and often a very vehement response.

There may be a gender influence here with stereotyped ideas linking nursing with housewifery and some male/female differences. Male doctors were less likely to tidy up after themselves than female, although there were some male doctors who did so. The senior house officer and junior registrar level is where there is most doctor irritation. Consultants are not expected to clear up after treatments, medical students and house officers almost invariably are, so registrar and SHO irritation can be seen as relating to their position in the medical structure.

An important aspect of tidying concerns the nature of clinical debris. All nurses and doctors agreed that doctors should tidy up 'sharps' (i.e. objects such as needles and scalpels), but it was evident that practice did not always match agreed policy. Some nurses were resigned to general tidying, but they too were angry when doctors did not tidy away 'sharps', and left them lying on the patient's bed or locker. This was universally condemned – though it still happened – because of the risks to the patient, and to ward and laundry staff of being cut, and infected (i.e. hepatitis, AIDS).

Individual nurses are not always consistent: 'I'll do it if they ask nicely and they are busy and I am not', or if doctor X is an especially popular or considerate person who is generally helpful. One in five nurses said they would tidy up after a doctor providing this was not taken for granted by doctors, a response that suggests that the issue here is not one of extra work, but a sense of professional pride. In practice there is some inconsistency because the workload of junior doctors and staff nurses varies so widely. Staff who can recognise that colleagues are exhausted and make adjustments to normal practice are much appreciated, but risk being left to clear up on other occasions also. The variety of attitudes means that a doctor, whose work takes him or her on and off wards all the time, may well be able to evade responsibility, and will frequently try to do so. In the end many nurses do tidy up after doctors, but resent doing so, and take refuge in continuous nagging which is often ignored.

The situation where the question of tidying blows up into a major conflict is when cleaning staff are not available and trained nursing staff find themselves expected to clear away dishes and mugs that doctors have left behind. This was reported as a rare event, but one that was more likely to happen as a result of cleaners' duties being narrowly defined following competitive tendering of cleaning contracts. Nurses do not have such tightly defined contracts.

In one hospital there was a clear hospital policy that defined responsibility for tidying clinical debris, but this was often unknown to doctors. These quotes are from the same ward team where there was claimed to be an agreed policy that doctors should tidy up after themselves.

> *Sister*: If a doctor makes a mess and leaves the trolley. . . I will bleep them and if they don't come back and clear it up I will get the Registrar . . . Bad manners aren't lost when they get to medical school.

> *Consultant*: If the nurses are going to abrogate their responsibility for tidying up as well, then one really quite wonders what they are supposed to do.

(iii) Nurse manager–doctor conflict

Accounts of conflict or anger that involved nurse managers were most commonly made by consultants and senior registrars and gave the clearest evidence of competing professions.

Nurse managers typically have responsibility for several wards, often belonging to two or three different specialties. They are responsible for managing the nursing staff budget, the largest single item of cost for most departments. Both the nurse manager and the ward nurse belong to the same profession, are part of the same line management structure, are guided by the same professional rules. At the same time, it is the consultant who is concerned with the treatment of the patients on the ward, and on some wards the consultant works more closely with the ward nursing staff than does the nurse manager. Nurse managers are responsible for the ward nursing staff, but consultants also see the nurses on their ward as 'their' nurses, part of the natural nurse–doctor clinical team. So there is some tussling for influence and authority.

> *Consultant*: Nursing management always makes me mad. Certain members of nursing management have commented to nurses on the ward 'You shouldn't be talking to doctors about that, that's a nursing thing' . . . it is almost as if they are trying to engender mistrust between the two groups.

> *Nurse manager*: I was desperately trying to get the nurses to develop their skills, and not just stay in one theatre . . . so I made a rota and started to move, and the people the nurses went to complain to were the consultants . . . I went to the sister and said 'It makes me very sad that the nurse can't go through her own group to me, she has got to go to that profession.' Because I still think that some of the nursing profession feel that the doctors are their boss, and that I'm not.

The number of consultants working in a nurse manager's area ranged from two to 20. Many of the doctors interviewed were critical of some aspect of nursing management, though the number of incidents of overt conflict was not high. This may be partly explained by the limited contact there is between nurse managers and medical staff; a third of the nurse managers interviewed said that they had little contact with either consultants or junior doctors. Both consultants and nurse managers varied in the time that they spent on wards.

Ward sisters have divided responsibilities (Figure 2.2). The patients on the ward are the responsibility of the consultant and the sister is responsible to the consultant for their care, but the consultant is not her line manager. Ward sisters are appointed by nurse managers and are accountable to them for the management of nursing staff and the quality of nursing care. A ward sister is therefore accountable both to the consultant and also to the nurse manager. Some of the criticisms made of nurse managers related to their unenviable responsibility for ensuring that all the wards in their control were adequately staffed with the right mix of nurses at different grades. This is discussed in Chapter 4.

Nurse managers confront the consultant at times, sometimes because of the behaviour of consultants, or the incompetence of junior doctors, or to press for organisational changes that are thought likely to benefit patients. Consultants seek to influence the decisions of nurse managers if this is likely to improve nurse staffing levels for their ward, but generally try to limit the control of nurse managers, unless they are involved with the clinical care of patients, as some are.

Both nurse managers and senior medical staff claimed that the other group had to be ignored at times because they were insufficiently innovative, and would be a barrier to necessary change if they were consulted. For nurse managers this was exemplified by the attitude of some consultants to the introduction of team nursing or primary nursing; for consultants it was demonstrated by the fact that nurse managers did not keep up to date with new medical treatments. Both were stressing the priority each gave to the area of hospital life for which each was responsible; patient care for nurse managers, patient treatment for medical staff.

Primary nursing means that a named nurse is responsible for the care of a very small number of patients, who continue to be the responsibility of the same nurse until they are discharged. Team nursing is a variant of this system. One of the implications of primary nursing is that it takes away the hierarchical nature of the ward organisation. For the doctor it means that there is not just one single person who will know the state of health of all the patients on the ward. The decision to implement this new style of nursing organisation is usually taken by the ward sister and nursing officer

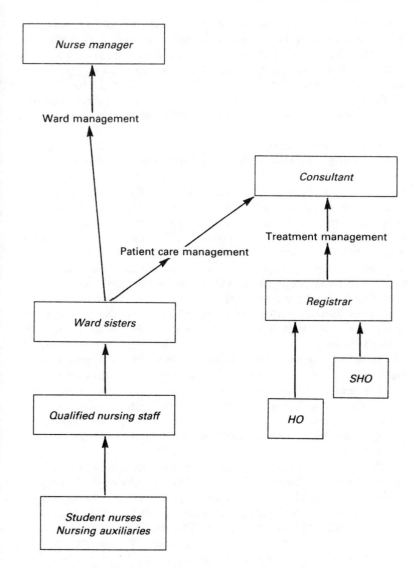

Figure 2.2 *Ward accountability*

together, and usually involves some discussion with the unit general manager because there are staffing implications. A move to primary nursing will also normally be discussed with the consultants who are based on the ward, but sometimes this will be perfunctory, especially if they are infrequently on the ward or if they have an autocratic style. A consultant may find that 'his or her' ward has been reorganised, or is going to be reorganised, without the consultant being fully involved in the decision. On one site we were informed that the doctors had not been involved in discussions specifically because it was known that they would try to block the implementation of such policy. Other hospitals were discussing with medical staff what this would mean in terms of the exchange of information.

An area of contention from a consultant's viewpoint is the process of appointing ward sisters. At one time a consultant would have had a dominant say in who was selected for this pivotal responsibility on 'his/her' ward. That has not been the case for several years, but consultants who commented were convinced that they should be able to control, or at least significantly influence, the appointment of ward sisters. For the nursing profession, control of these appointments is absolutely fundamental to the notion of nursing as an independent profession. While consultant resentment was present in most hospitals, it was in the two Scottish hospitals that consultants were pressing their case most vigorously. Nurse managers varied in the extent to which they would allow any consultant involvement in the selection process, from no involve-ment, to sitting in on interviews but not having a veto. Our sample of nurse managers commenting on this was too small to be statistically significant. However, our impression was that medical involvement in nursing interviews is one of the few conflict issues where there was a gender factor, with male nurse managers more strongly opposed to consultant involvement of any kind. The creation of clinical directorates, led by a doctor, is likely to re-open this controversy.

When clinical directorates are formed a decision has to be made as to who should have responsibility for the nursing budget for the directorate. Usually this is the nurse manager. In one of the five hospitals used for interviews there was a possibility that the medical director would control this budget. This kind of situation is a clear example of the way that devolving budgets leads to changing patterns of interprofessional relations. Discussion of clinical bud-gets is continued in Chapter 5.

Nursing practice has to be consistent with the code of professional conduct issued by nursing's controlling body, the United Kingdom Central Council for Nursing, Midwifery and Health Visiting (UKCC). Nurse managers have to ensure that nursing practice in their unit and hospital is consistent with the code, and the other guidelines issued by the UKCC. There are also policy documents and protocols agreed within the hospital, or the health authority, that have to be implemented and monitored. Junior doctors are acutely aware that nurses work to rules that determine the nature and limits of their professional responsibilities, but that these are linked to national guidelines is less well understood. A widespread belief among junior doctors is that nurses are restricted by the policies laid down by local nurse managers. Particular incidents varied widely, but the statement that nurses are too rigid in the application of rules was frequently repeated.

This is related to the way that nurses are authorised to take responsibility for additional tasks through a system of 'extended role' certification for specific tasks. When doctors comment on nursing rigidity they are often essentially criticising the extended role system and a concept of professionalism that emphasises rules rather than autonomous judgement. On this issue the nursing profession, through its governing body, the UKCC, decided in July 1992 that criticism of the extended role system had been justified, and professional regulations have been changed (see Chapter 3).

(iv) Doctor–doctor conflict

At times nurses find themselves embroiled in arguments that are essentially intra-medical rather than interprofessional. Almost all accounts concerned consultants; disputes between more junior medical staff were only of passing interest. Most were given by nursing staff from theatres and intensive care units (ICUs), with few from ward staff. This was one of the very few areas where medical staff were not willing to give comment in any detail. Most accounts involved questions of control over the treatment agenda of patients in intensive care, or establishing priorities in the use of limited theatre facilities. In these situations nursing staff could be caught in the crossfire, or expected to settle conflicting claims.

These incidents raise some interesting questions. Does conflict between consultants create a space which nurses use to extend their own influence, or is such conflict a burden that nursing staff regret? And are such disputes settled by reference to professional status and hierarchy, or to patient well-being?

The unit would usually have a consultant anaesthetist, a registrar and a senior house officer, though in some units there were two registrars. The consultant on ICU has specialist knowledge of the techniques and treatment necessary to maintain life, and to control pain, and it is this consultant who routinely supervises patient care in ICU. The patient, though, remains the responsibility of the consultant to whom he or she had been initially referred for hospital admission. To use a phrase often quoted to us, the admitting consultant 'owns' the patient. The way that this dual responsibility is handled varied considerably, not only between different hospitals, but also between consultants.

In two of the district hospitals this division of responsibilities had not caused difficulties. ICU consultants implied that they would expect their advice to be accepted. In one of the teaching hospitals there had been problems in the past, and a clear protocol existed confirming that the final say was with the admitting consultant. The protocol was based on the prior claim of the admitting consultant, and not on an independent assessment of the patient's needs. Nurses expressed anger at the attitude of a consultant who would not accept the expertise of the ICU consultant on the management of pain relief, in a way that they felt was to the detriment of patient care, but accepted that they could not query the decision. Careful questioning suggested that while this had happened it was not a common event. More commonly, the 'visiting' consultant will insist on maintaining treatment when the unit nursing staff are convinced that there is no hope, and nurses feel that this view is shared, if not stated, by the ICU consultant. Authority is again vested in the consultant's professional 'ownership' of the patient. At one of the district hospitals aspects of ICU management were causing tensions at the time of the interviews, but there was no indication that nursing staff regarded consultant conflict as anything but an irritation that had to be accepted.

> *Staff nurse*: The surgeons want one thing for their patients, and the anaesthetist who's looking after the patient in ICU might want something else . . . and the medics and the anaesthetists very much resent each other . . . but it doesn't tend to affect us much. I mean, it's noticeable, but the patients still get their care.

To return to the questions that we posed earlier, the evidence from ICU is that nurses do not in any way use conflict between consultants as an opportunity to extend their influence. The situation was regretted, sometimes bitterly, but accepted as being outside their sphere of influence.

Operating theatres are booked to surgeons at specific times of the week, with emergency theatre facilities available at other times. Anaesthetists have rotas to cover all the theatres in the district, which will often be at more than one hospital. Theatre sisters usually manage a suite of theatres at any one hospital. In staffing theatres, anaesthetists have to be managers of an expensive facility spread over many sites, while surgeons are concerned with the particular patient they want to treat at that time. Some disagreement between surgeons and anaesthetists is inevitable. Nurses tend to be primarily spectators of such conflicts.

A different situation arises with emergency theatre. When emergency cases go to theatre there may be more than one surgeon wanting access to theatre at the same time. The ideal would be a dispassionate assessment of relative patient need, but in practice this does not happen. Both the anaesthetists and the theatre nursing staff may find themselves in the centre of disputes between surgeons over access to theatre. A theatre sister who valued diplomacy highly told us with some embarrassment why she had lost her temper with a medical colleague.

> *Theatre sister*: They all see their patient as the one with priority, and they tend to off-load the decision of who goes into the [emergency] theatre first onto the nurse in charge of the theatre . . . It was a situation like that where I wouldn't take on the responsibility of saying who was going first and one surgeon said that all the nursing staff in this theatre were totally incompetent. I just saw red.

As in ICU, there is no evidence that nurses use disputes between doctors to extend their influence. Theatre sisters are usually detached observers, or actively refuse to accept responsibility for rationing the use of theatre time by different consultants.

If there is a clear protocol to determine which consultant has authority, nursing staff accept the protocol. This is the situation in some intensive care units. These rules are linked to the admitting consultant's position as the person who 'owns' the patient. They are not settled by any assessment of patient-based criteria. Nursing staff may urge consultants to settle disputes, but they do not challenge the consultants' authority to settle the matter.

Contested authority: a summary

This section has looked at the evidence of conflict between medical and nursing staff over the exercise of professional authority in hospital wards. The consultant's authority over treatment was evident throughout all accounts. Nursing staff contested the decisions of junior medical staff, but usually by reference to usual practice on the ward, thereby generally enforcing senior medical staff authority.

The balance of authority between nurses and more junior medical staff is more varied. There is resentment that nursing observations are ignored by doctors, and irritation when nursing staff do not communicate relevant information. The relative status of both groups is uncertain, and task priorities have to be negotiated, though responsibilities for tasks are usually tightly defined. Nurses are increasingly refusing to act as 'handmaidens', but in practice many do accept responsibility for mundane tasks such as tidying up.

Pressure to reduce junior doctor hours has led to a reassessment of some responsibilities. Some nursing staff judge whether they should accept responsibilities by reference to patients' interests, but there is an awareness that tasks may be 'dumped' on nursing staff. The nursing profession has formally moved away from the process of certification for precise tasks, but the cultural values that underpinned this process remain strong. There is a strong sense of hierarchical professional control in nursing, though the introduction of primary nursing may encourage the devolution of authority down to the nurse responsible for a patient's care. Where there is conflict between medical staff, nursing staff are likely to ignore what is happening if this is possible.

A different area of tension is between consultants and nurse managers. The organisation of nursing services on a ward is not controlled by consultants, but consultants who interest themselves in nursing issues are likely to be involved in discussions. Consultants see it as entirely appropriate that they should have a significant say in the appointment of senior ward nursing staff, but this is a matter of considerable symbolic and practical significance to nursing staff, particularly nurse managers. Cultural differences between the professions lead to different concepts of professional behaviour, and this difference underpins some conflict.

B: CARE OR TREATMENT?

In discussions with medical and nursing staff, caring for patients and treating patients were commonly described as if these were distinctive processes, the first being a nursing responsibility, the latter a medical one. The boundary between them is determined by a mix of traditional working practices, the nature of the task, and the skill, experience and authority of individual practitioners. Authority to settle disputes over the location of the boundary is contested, as previously discussed, but here there is a different factor. For some nurses this boundary helps to define what constitutes nursing as a distinctive process, so that determining the location of the boundary and defending it has symbolic importance. The nature of acute hospital care is constantly changing, so that the boundary has to be periodically re-negotiated, thus giving rise to episodic demarcation disputes. Even when there is agreement as to what constitutes care or treatment, there are still issues of which take precedence.

A shifting boundary   There are numerous examples of shifting boundaries: IV drug administration has already been discussed. Other areas are intensive care, the treatment of terminally ill patients, the management of wounds, and the development of triage systems in accident and emergency departments. A specific example of shifting boundaries is control of elimination (bowel and bladder emptying), which is one of the areas generally recognised as being managed by nurses. On one of the wards we visited the ward sister had just had an energetic exchange with the consultant over his practice of carrying out a bowel examination (a PR, or per rectal) on elderly patients during every ward round.

> *Ward sister*: I feel really that doctors are taking on too much of what I consider to be nursing roles . . . and that annoys me. For instance, the things that have been happening recently is them doing PRs on the ward round . . . that's disgusting, and plus the fact it was making the ward rounds take until about 6 o'clock in the evening, we just haven't got the time . . . I'm just not going to let that happen again.

That two groups of professional staff who are both under heavy work pressure should be in conflict over the management of elimination may seem on the surface surprising, but particular tasks are the raw material through which professional territories are partly defined. The movement of such boundaries indicates shifting patterns of territorial authority.

In the example above, the ward sister was resenting what she saw as an invasion of medical staff into her professional area, while the consultant was claiming a right to ensure that he was able to assess the health of patients for whom he was legally responsible. In discussion of IV drug administration there was a different aspect evident, in that some nursing staff saw it as an attempt to dump on them tasks that doctors wanted to discard, and were therefore resisting responsibility for IV drug administration (treatment), though they accepted that oral drug administration (care) was their responsibility.

Intensive care   A different pattern is evident in intensive care units. Patients in ICU are likely to have come from very complex surgery, to have experienced severe trauma, or to have liver or kidney failure. Many patients will be on a ventilator, a machine which takes over and controls the patient's breathing. Most will have IV drips, and be fed either through nasal tube or IV drip. There is constant monitoring of body fluids, blood pressure, and blood gas level. ICU nurses are highly trained, often with formal post-registration certification, and with their expertise acknowledged by the departmental consultant and other doctors.

In ICU nurses have developed skills and accept responsibility for areas of treatment management that at one time would have been unquestionably within a medical domain. Consultants in ICU support the development of nursing skills, and set parameters within which nurses will decide on levels of sedation, or assess change in ways that appear strikingly similar to making a diagnosis, but this is perceived as part of a process of providing care.

Wound management   Wound management is an area where some of the features of a confused care–treatment boundary are most evident. Wound healing requires considerable expertise, particularly pressure sores: it is essential to relieve pressure on the wound; if an ulcer is compressed between the bone and the bed it will not heal. A reasonable level of health is needed for rapid wound healing; if people are malnourished this process will take a long time. A crucial task is to stop the wound becoming infected, or to clean up existing infection without destroying more tissue.

There is a division of labour between doctors and nurses on wounds. The nurses characteristically decide what they will use for the wound. However, a prescription and a doctor's signature will be needed in certain circumstances, for instance, if the wound is very complex, such as a severe open pressure sore, and needs to be treated with specialised wound care material. In very severe cases, plastic surgery is required. At this end of the spectrum it is uncontentious that it is a doctor's responsibility. There is therefore a gradation between wounds involving doctors, such as those needing plastic surgery, and those which are accepted as being within a nursing remit, such as small pressure sores. In between, there may be points where the doctor will say that one course of action is needed and the nurse says something different.

Of the different kinds of wounds, surgical incisions heal with least difficulty, while promoting the healing of pressure sores and ulcers can be extremely difficult and require much skill. A division of professional responsibility based on greater knowledge of the physiology of healing would suggest that nurses would manage the dressings of surgical incisions while doctors controlled the treatment of pressure sores, or that nurses would be reluctant holders of responsibility for dealing with complex pressure sores. Both assumptions are incorrect. A few doctors insist on their right to decide on the best treatment of pressure sores, but this is usually fiercely contested by nurses who see the management of pressure sores as being firmly within their sphere of control, so that the doctor is expected to listen to nursing advice when obliged to write the prescription for dressings that can only be written by a doctor. Some doctors refuse to accept nursing advice. A consultant reported conflict on a surgical unit:

Consultant: There is a doctor who has got some correspondence going with one of the sisters on the ward who will not use the sort of wound care that he likes and she says that it is the nurse's responsibility what sort of wound care she uses and he says that she should use the wound care that he prescribes.

Interviewer: Is there a right on either side?

Consultant: I think that it is the responsibility of the nurses to do what is prescribed by the doctor because he is legally responsible for the care of that patient. But if you talk to the Chief Nursing Officer he would say that the nurse must do what she feels is right and take the consequences if she feels that she is doing it correctly, so I suppose both sides of the profession listen to their professional advisers and that's where the line is drawn. I think it is viewed on the medical side as being the tip of the iceberg. I think what is going to happen in these particular circumstances is that the consultants will actually actively prescribe wound care in the future and it will come slightly like the American system where you prescribe the diet and everything else.

Doctors rarely intervene in pressure sore management despite their greater complexity and obduracy, since their cause is related to nursing issues. The healing of pressure sores can only be achieved if patients are frequently turned, or helped to become mobile, and, in some cases, if continence is achieved. These tasks are nursing responsibilities that no doctor we met had any desire to claim.

This increasing interest by doctors in wounds may be related to the fact that wound treatment is an area in which there is a development of research. Wound healing is therefore an area of expertise where nurses justify their claim to control care by reference to scientific knowledge and practical experience, precisely the same criteria that medicine uses to justify its status. We found that some doctors would listen to nursing research, others had to be approached 'diplomatically' if nursing staff were to succeed in having their prescription choice agreed, and a small number of doctors flatly refused to look at research papers, or listen to the views of nursing staff. In these situations the hierarchical control of medicine was imposed.

Intervention in the care of dying patients   Questions about the care of dying patients cannot easily be settled by reference to patient well-being, since all those concerned will argue that they are promoting the choice that is in the best interests of the patient. So when the needs of treatment and care conflict, how are decisions reached? Does treatment by doctors always take precedence over care by nurses, and who decides?

Disagreement over the treatment of terminally ill patients was raised spontaneously and quite frequently by nurses. If a patient is clearly dying there are judgement calls over the balance between the quality of life and the extent of the prolongation of life. Examples of this include the question of whether to use pain-killers that do not cause death but may speed the process of dying; when it is justified to undertake painful invasive investigations with a low likelihood of success; in what circumstances to mark a patient's notes as 'not for resuscitation'; and when a decision should be taken to turn off a life-support machine. All of these questions involve ethical issues. The aim here is restricted to giving an accurate and representative account of issues raised by staff.

Modern pain-killers can be effective against extreme forms of pain. However, in large doses they may reduce the chance of living longer. So should diamorphine be given at levels that are known to speed death, when that level is necessary in order to relieve pain? The question presents in its most acute form when a house officer or SHO is called out to see an emergency at night:

> *SHO*: Very often nurses will want to instigate end stage treatment very much earlier than the doctors would . . . particularly say at weekends or on call overnight if somebody is admitted and they're obviously distressed . . . the nurses will try and get the junior house officer to instigate diamorphine infusions and . . . it can be a source of conflict if the doctor is not willing to take that step.

Further investigations may have a chance of being medically useful, but they may be invasive and painful. There is a decision as to the extent to which new drug treatments or invasive investigations are justified when the patient is clearly, or very probably, dying. The problem is that they may be painful, or have very unpleasant side effects. They disrupt the patient that the nurses are trying to make comfortable.

> *Staff nurse*: At the end . . . the houseman was discussing all the things that he wanted to have done, like the ECG and the X-ray and everything, and I said, 'Can I ask why? Because if it was my grandfather, I would not like him to be treated in this way. Why can't we just . . . give him pain-killers and let him die . . . you know he's got cancer everywhere . . .' The houseman said to the consultant 'well . . . are you going to stick up for the nurses or stick up for the doctor?' And the consultant went through the different things and said [they were] unnecessary.

A closely related issue is whether and, if so, when a patient should be declared 'not for resuscitation'. This may be written into the notes so that if there is a heart attack the coronary arrest team is not called to revive them.

Staff nurse: [the decision] not to send out a call is usually the registrar's
. . . it depends how ill the person is . . . If it is someone who has been
in the ward for a while and they are very ill, we discuss it, we would
probably say look do you really want us to put out a call for this lady?
And normally they say no.

Intervention is not an issue on some wards: it is the consultant's
decision but he or she does take the views of the nursing staff into
account.

Intense disagreement can occur when a patient is dying after a
major operation. Death is evidence of the failure of surgery, and
surgeons may have a very strong commitment to carry on trying to
maintain life while other staff see death as inevitable. On some
wards junior doctors reported that, while in theory all the staff
closely involved are consulted before a decision is taken to end
treatment, in practice the consultant never asks anyone. The levels
of conflict are reduced if there is a willingness to take the opinion of
colleagues into account. This depends on individuals at least as
much as on policy.

The decision to cease treatment in the case of terminally ill
patients is a conflict which involves not only the issues of hierarchy,
and that of the diagnosis–care boundary, but also that of the
differing philosophies over preserving life at any cost versus the
significance of the quality of life. Individual doctors and nurses have
strong and sometimes divergent views.

Care or treatment: a summary

Nursing and medical staff refer to 'care' as a process distinct from
'treatment'. To researchers, the distinctions between care and
treatment appeared at times to have a historical base rather than a
functional one, and the boundary between them is confused and
constantly changing. It is a boundary along which territorial disputes are sometimes conducted, at times demonstrating aspects of
professional organisation that are not compatible with the notion of
flexible interprofessional teamwork.

Disagreements are compounded by the fact that important
aspects of care, generally a nursing domain, can only be implemented through the prescription of suitable drugs, which is a
medical responsibility. The reverse is true also; the provision of
drug treatment by doctors is largely dependent on the administration of drugs by nurses. In hospital, neither care nor treatment
can be provided by a profession acting alone.

Wound dressing provides some examples of conflict over whether
there is a hierarchy which is mediated through the treatment–care
boundary. This boundary is necessarily fuzzy in practice, although

in abstract it sounds very plausible. At some points the nurse's function of caring demands so much skill and contains so much expertise that it effectively crosses over into treatment, and having crossed this divide, doctors may seek to reclaim control. Since most wound management requires prescriptions, and prescriptions in hospital are issued by doctors, medical staff are able to claim control if they wish to do so.

Intensive care staff locate the care–treatment boundary very differently. Medical staff are dependent on nurses extending their responsibility into areas previously considered to be medical. Nevertheless, in the actions of ICU consultants who seek to extend nursing roles, and of those consultants who stress their authority to decide on wound management, the common theme is control of the agenda by medical staff. This does not imply inevitable nursing dissent, since consultant authority, as was shown earlier, is accepted by nursing staff in most situations.

Different values surface in the process of responding to the needs of dying patients. To return to a question we posed earlier, treatment does not always take precedence over care, and care of dying patients, as opposed to treatment, is valued by doctors as well as by nursing staff. A theoretical position that ascribes 'care' exclusively to nurses is as misleading as one that claims all 'treatment' to be medical. It was noticeable that two of the areas where there was most tension over the care–treatment boundary involved less pleasant aspects of nursing care: elimination and pressure sore management. Nursing appears to have gained expertise in these areas because doctors have not been interested in their management.

The distinction between medical and nursing roles that appeared most evident, namely the contrast between the continual presence of nursing staff on a ward, and the episodic nature of medical ward visits, was only occasionally suggested as a way of defining the boundary between medicine and nursing. Yet there is an appealing logic in the notion that any form of care or treatment that has to be regularly or continuously provided for ill people is a form of nursing so that a workable boundary could be determined by the frequency with which treatment or care is required.

C: PATIENTS FIRST?

In examining medical–nursing boundary issues, what evidence is there that contentious issues are settled by reference to patients' interests? This is a question that is central to a discussion of the value of devolving autonomy downward to professional staff. If the boundaries between professions are settled by reference to professional interests or prestige, rather than patient well-being, then the value of professional autonomy is questionable.

Before looking at the range of issues raised in the study, there are two aspects of professional work that are particularly relevant: the question of how staff deal with evidence of inadequate care or treatment, and the level of concern for issues of dignity, privacy and respect for patients.

(i) Controlling bad practice

Looking at how nursing and medicine react to evidence of poor quality treatment shows the relative weight attached to concerns for patient well-being and for professional protection. If the patient comes 'first', as common rhetoric proclaims, then bad practice by the other profession can legitimately be challenged. If, conversely, the maintenance of professional boundaries takes precedence, it is a reasonable judgement that 'patients first' is more of a slogan than an ethic. This is a substantial area of debate; our evidence is limited but has the value of being rooted in ward-based interactions.

We found that where a doctor is considered by the nursing staff to be incompetent or uncaring, the ward sister or staff nurse will challenge the doctor directly, and if that has no impact then the matter will be discussed with more senior medical colleagues. Ward sisters will make sure that the consultants are aware of consistent poor practice, either by speaking to them directly, or working through the registrar. If a particular incident is immediately threatening to a patient, such as a house officer or SHO refusing to turn out at night, or a registrar declaring an intention to carry out a treatment that the nursing staff are convinced is undesirable, then the consultant may be contacted at home. The nurse invokes the authority of the consultant in order to control a junior member of the medical staff.

One such incident, described to us by a nurse as being an 'irritation', involved a potential amputation and could scarcely have been more dramatic, though it was not typical of the accounts we were given. Typical accounts concerned registrars inadequately conducting a treatment procedure, house officers or SHOs being persistently slow to come when bleeped, or regularly failing to record patient information. The underlying feature was an individual seen as consistently providing poor quality work, or seriously disrupting ward routine.

There was plenty of evidence of nurses willingly crossing the professional divide to see that a doctor's incompetence was challenged. This reflects the disciplinary practices of nursing, which lay considerable stress on monitoring and accountability. It is resented by junior doctors who are shown up to senior medical colleagues as incompetent, and who share the cultural values of medicine, which stress individual responsibility.

When medical staff are regularly dissatisfied with the work of a staff nurse or other nursing staff their complaints are usually conveyed informally to the ward sister by the registrar or consultant. Often this is in connection with nursing duties that have an immediate bearing on medical work, for example, a nurse who cannot be relied on to see that fluid intake is measured accurately, or ward staff who fail to get patients ready for theatre when the surgeon is expecting them.

The exchanges we have just described are all 'in house'; the criticism has remained within the medical–nursing grouping that constitutes the ward team. Difficulties arise when the problem is the quality of the ward sister or consultant's work. When a consultant becomes concerned about the quality of patient care generally, or feels for whatever reason that the ward is not well managed, a decision has to be made as to whether to challenge the ward sister, with whom it is important to have a good relationship, or to opt for a peaceful if uneasy coexistence. A challenge to the ward sister necessitates moving marginally outside the ward team, which, as generally envisaged by medical staff, does not include the nurse manager (see Figure 2.2 on p. 35).

A formal complaint from a consultant to a nurse manager about a ward sister meant both crossing a professional divide, and acting against the grain of medical culture, with its stress on mutual support of professional colleagues. For some consultants this was not an easy decision. Patient care, as in this example, had to be undeniably bad before this step was taken.

> *Consultant (care of the elderly)*: The chap had been in hospital for a
> week and I introduced myself to him. I said hello, how was he getting
> on? He was quite well apart from the fact that he had an ulcer on his
> foot and none of the nurses knew about this ulcer . . . he had an ulcer
> on his foot with a patch of granuflex on it, which is a particular
> dressing which you usually change every three or four days and they
> didn't know about this . . . and that is how it manifested to me that
> they hadn't actually been bathing the patient . . . and the other
> circumstance that led me to . . . go further up the nursing manage-
> ment structure was when student nurses on the ward actually
> approached me in tears about the standard of care that some of the
> patients had got . . . you know, just unbelievable things, just very
> basic.

Where a consultant is felt to be remiss in either the quality of his/her work or attention to patient care it would require quite exceptional practice for nursing staff to initiate action. There would have to be evidence of serious malpractice, and the formal process of following through the criticism would require some courage. In practice, the disciplinary system required to examine consultant practice is triggered when there is a formal complaint from a patient. A consultant may go 'up the nursing management system' to have bad nursing practice investigated, but there is no equivalent medical hierarchy that a nurse can easily contact.

To put this into perspective, interviews were conducted in five health authority districts, and in many wards and departments. There was one ward in one hospital where three respondents, one medical and two nursing, on separate occasions and without prompting, expressed their unease about the consultant on their unit, but made clear that there would be no action.

The picture that emerges is that both doctors and nurses will cross professional boundaries relatively easily to discipline staff below the level of ward sister and consultant. A consultant may be reluctant to confront a ward sister whose work is inadequate, unless there is a formal complaint or action is initiated by nursing staff, and a challenge to a consultant's authority by the nursing staff is in practice an unlikely event.

Staff discipline is time consuming. A busy consultant may be unwilling to make the effort to discipline a more junior doctor whom he rarely sees. House officers and SHOs typically have contracts for six months. Even when a consultant is concerned the easy way out is to defer any action, knowing that the doctor will soon be leaving. The threat of a poor reference is the main disciplinary mechanism. The ward sister and the registrar may both be concerned about the quality of a junior doctor's work, or his/her disruptive influence on the ward, but if the doctor ignores them, and the consultant avoids confronting the issue there is a limit to their ability to change practice.

> *Senior registrar:* We have got a chap working here at the moment . . . the first day when I came back you could tell there were vibes . . . And then sister came to me later on and said this guy is just . . .!!, but . . . well this chap is actually quite clever because he plays the game, he keeps his nose clean with his seniors.

With nurses in permanent posts the easy option of waiting for them to leave is not available, and both the professional codes and the cultural attitudes within nursing are such that errors and deviations from accepted practice are more likely to be reported to senior nursing staff and formally dealt with through procedures involving written warnings, suspension and dismissal. Nevertheless, some incidents of poor nursing are not dealt with adequately

(Mackay, 1989). There is a significant difference in the way that nursing and junior medical staff are treated if an error occurs, and this is noted with irritation by nursing staff.

(ii) Lack of respect and courtesy to patients

There were 15 reports of conflicts generated by lack of respect and courtesy to patients, 13 of them from nurses. Doctors made comments indicating that they saw nurses behaving in ways that were insensitive, but these observations were not linked to conflict. Medical staff do not appear to think it appropriate to comment to colleagues on their behaviour to patients.

Contemporary nursing theory emphasises the position of the patient as an individual within the family, and care that is holistic and extends to relatives. This is markedly different from what is sometimes scornfully dismissed as the medical model which is focused on the treatment of disease. A nurse who is outspoken in his/her concern for a patient's dignity can generate conflict with a doctor. Some nurses will take a doctor aside and reveal their feelings very strongly if they feel a patient has been distressed in any way by a doctor's attitude. If necessary, they will confront the doctor in public.

> *Staff nurse*: [The professor] was doing a teaching round and there were about 10 medical students with him, and a junior nurse came up to me and said 'they are teaching and the man is sitting on a commode.' I looked around, they had pulled the curtain back, the man was sitting on a commode, an old frail man, I think he was oblivious to what was going on really, but it doesn't matter, and there were these 10 students and the professor, and I was so angry that they could do that that I had to go up to him and say 'Excuse me, professor, but would you mind not doing that just now.'

Wards and departments where there is a strong teaching commitment generate conflicts over whether patients should take part in teaching sessions, particularly when nursing staff feel that this is too stressful for a patient who is very ill or frail. There is a cultural difference in the value placed on teaching and research by nurses and by doctors.

A recurrent theme is that senior doctors are uniquely pressured, and their work must always take precedence. A consultant who was about to interrupt a visit from the chaplain to a seriously ill patient was furious when the sister insisted this should not happen. He could see no reason why he should not take precedence. In general, though, doctors do accept that it is reasonable for nurses to remind them of the need for courtesy and respect, and recognise that the pressures on them do mean that at times they ignore patients' feelings. Sometimes the doctor's response seems to be one of surprise and dismay that he/she has upset a patient.

> *Senior registrar*: One thing I am weak on is recognising the emotional implications . . . I like to feel I can work out how [patients] take us, but you do miss it sometimes, and you have a situation they will find horrific . . . and you miss it, and that does upset me.

Patients first: a summary

The question was asked earlier if staff appear to settle disputes by any reference to patient interests or objective assessment of potential outcomes. A related issue is whether confrontation is avoided when it is necessary to confront poor quality or potentially damaging treatment or care.

Patient well-being took precedence over respect for the maintenance of professional boundaries when the disciplining of junior medical and nursing staff was necessary, but there was some degree of reluctance on the part of senior medical staff in confronting poor practice on the part of ward sisters, and patient well-being would normally be seriously at risk before formal complaints were made. Consultant authority is justified by status, backed by his/her position as the person to whom the patient has been referred. On the very rare occasions when concern was expressed about the commitment or competence of a consultant there was no challenge to his/her authority from nursing or junior medical staff.

Issues of dignity and respect are afforded a much higher status in nursing philosophy than in medicine where the emphasis is on diagnosis and cure, though this does not imply that individual doctors ignore such concerns. Doctors generally accepted that it was legitimate for nurses to remind them that their behaviour to patients was lacking in courtesy, providing that this was done diplomatically. There was doubt as to whether this would lead to changed practice. A degree of scepticism was also at times expressed by doctors as to whether nurses as a profession were the correct people to act as the patient's advocate when nurses' behaviour could also show a lack of sensitivity on occasion. In defending the right of patients to be treated with respect nurses are sometimes assertive in a way that is not always true where their own interests are concerned.

Rules for the administration of medicines was an area of clinical work where it was very clear that patient well-being has precedence over respect for professional status and boundaries, but in deciding who should be responsible for the administration of IV drugs there was less clarity. For some staff, IV drug administration was influenced by considering the immediate impact on patient care, but this was not a universal position.

Disputes over the boundary of care and treatment were as likely to be settled by referring to the legal responsibility of the consultant as they were by a dispassionate assessment of the relative value for a patient of different treatment processes. Patient well-being may have primacy when a procedure is established, but does not appear to be an accepted criterion for determining the allocation of task responsibilities.

Different professions: a conflict theme

During interviews there were times when both nurses and doctors discussed in some detail what it meant to them to be a professional. What was striking was that the concept of being a professional for a doctor was such a different notion in practice to what a nurse meant by being a professional. It is the underlying feature of many of the intense irritations expressed by doctors about nursing practices. The issue at stake is whether a profession consists of individuals who make decisions and act on their judgement, or a body of people who constantly monitor their practice and standards. To many nurses a professional is someone accountable for their practice, guided by rules, and monitored by senior professionals. Rules are annoying at times, but protect nurses from legal challenge and provide security when work involves many stressful situations. To a doctor, a professional is someone who will take responsibility for his/her own judgements and actions, so detailed rules can appear as unprofessional restrictions. Doctors often think that nurses do not take responsibility, while nurses often think that doctors get away with levels of slipshod practice that would be unacceptable in nursing.

If the work of the two professions was unrelated, the existence of two different cultural attitudes could continue without conflict, but because their work is so interdependent, differences in professional culture make some argument inevitable. These contrasting modes of operation are all the more interesting in that a directive from the UKCC (1992c: 2) states that 'practice must be based upon a set of sound principles rather than upon certificates for specific tasks'. The nursing profession is moving nearer to the medical concept of an autonomous individual – just as medicine, in accepting medical audit, is moving marginally nearer to nursing notions of accountability. However, there is no indication that nursing is any less resolved to have clear guidelines and monitoring of practitioners, rather a sense that the individual and not the profession is responsible for extending the nurse's practice while still working within a professional code. Nor is there an indication that doctors will be easily persuaded of the value of a more 'managerial' approach to professional regulation. Even so, moving away from an extended role certification system is a significant cultural change, as medical audit is for the medical profession.

Conclusion

The process of devolving authority downwards in hospitals to the staff who provide care means that aspects of professional authority is weakened, in so far as this is expressed through hierarchical structures, and interprofessional teams evolve their own decision making processes. In examining accounts of medical–nursing conflict we looked at how authority is currently negotiated, in order to see how systems of devolved authority might function. The distinction between care and treatment was examined to see whether this gave a clear basis for deciding how to allocate responsibilities. The extent to which patients interests were a defining criteria was also examined.

A distinction between 'caring' and 'treating' does not appear to be a sufficiently clear boundary to carry the weight of differentiating between two professions. It is an area where territorial disputes are visible. In some areas nursing expertise is such that nurses' work involves skills akin to those required in making a diagnosis and deciding on treatment. This is acceptable to doctors providing nurses are working for 'their' patients, within limits set by doctors, and within a team structure led by doctors, but nurses do not always accept these boundaries.

At the point of service provision nursing and medicine are both symbiotic and hierarchical in aspects of their relationship. Each needs the other to some extent, though this varies significantly in different areas of work. Medical staff have a more significant role in acute specialties than they have, for example, in the rehabilitation or long-term care of frail elderly patients. Medical and nursing staff operate in overlapping spheres that are independent of each other in part, and both hierarchical and interdependent in other aspects. Nursing staff emphasise the need for accountability to different people for different areas of responsibility. Medical staff see a need to control nursing so that a medical agenda has priority.

In so far as they are administering treatment, nurses are finally accountable to the consultant for the care of individual patients. Doctors below the level of consultant are also accountable to the consultant. This does not remove the requirement on either a nurse or a junior doctor to consider for themselves whether the actions they undertake constitute safe practice for the patient.

The consultant and the senior ward nursing staff are usually on permanent contracts, while more junior doctors are frequently on very short contracts. This can create loyalties that cut across professional divides. Nursing staff may influence the work of more junior doctors by referring to the consultant if junior medical staff make decisions that are considered unsafe, or incompatible with normal ward practice. In these situations they are acting as a proxy for the consultant.

The essential difference in the balance of power between the two professions lies in the consultant's ultimate responsibility for the patient in hospital, and the GP's responsibility for patient treatment outside hospital. This is expressed in a phrase we heard quite frequently; the consultant 'owns' the patient, an aspect of medical control that was not contested by any nurse in our study. Consultants are responsible for patients, and this sets a boundary to the extent of nursing influence within hospital. A junior doctor is moving toward this responsibility in training to become either a GP or a consultant. A nurse, however skilled, does not currently have 'ownership' of any hospital patients, though midwives may in the future do so (Department of Health, 1993).

For nurses and doctors to perform to their own satisfaction they need to have skilled colleagues. There is self-interest in seeing each group become more skilled, providing that this does not lead to challenges to existing authority. Neither profession wants to limit the skill of the other, though doctors do seek to control the skills of nurses so as to support their professional agenda, and nurses define the boundaries of their responsibility carefully so as to resist the extension of medical control. We found little evidence of nurses seeking to move into a medical area of influence, but there was resistance to taking over tasks that doctors wished to relinquish.

So there are separate spheres of influence, and contested ones. There is competition in protecting spheres of influence, but not in downgrading the work of the other profession, or in limiting the other's ability to gain more expertise in order to provide care or treatment more effectively. The more contentious issues are not related to the acquisition of skills, but to maintaining professional spheres of interest, and controlling priorities for the use of scarce resources of time, staff and budgets.

The area where we have seen most medical unease over loss of territory is in doctors' interaction with nurse managers, their inability fully to control how the ward is organised, and their inability to determine what nurses are allowed to do. Some nurses have asserted their control over aspects of ward organisation in establishing primary nursing systems in spite of medical disapproval. This has legitimacy because it is seen to be promoting patient well-being, and is supported by government directives. Patients' interests were seen to take precedence over the maintenance of professional boundaries in some, but not all, areas of tension.

The cultural values of medicine were seen to stress practitioner autonomy, while nursing emphasised adherence to rules. The process of devolving authority would seem to require adjustments to nursing attitudes if individual nurses are to accept responsibility for deciding their practice in line with recent UKCC guidance. Medical staff have to adjust to a greater surveillance of their work through audit and evaluation. In some respects, therefore, the cultural values of the two professions appear to be moving marginally closer.

The conflict accounts that have been examined so far have taken little account of health service changes. Other disagreements, some more intense, come from pressure on resources, and the difficulty of maintaining professional cooperation when ward teams are, at times, fragmented. These are examined in Chapter 4.

Our conclusions are based on the empirical evidence of a research study. How well they fit into theories of professions is the subject of the next chapter.

3

Interprofessional Relations in Theory and History

The day-to-day tensions in the working relations of doctors and nurses which were elaborated in the previous chapter will here be placed in the broader contexts of the theorisation of professions and of their historical development. How do we understand both the presence and absence of competition and friction between the professions in the light of theories of interprofessional conduct? How does the current balance of hierarchy and complementarity relate to previous patterns?

The struggle of occupations to become professions and reap the rewards of such a status is a major theme of the contemporary literature on the sociology of professions. Medicine has often been taken as the prime example of a successful profession, while nursing is seen as not yet having obtained this status. Is this the best way of understanding interprofessional relations between doctors and nurses in NHS hospitals today? Does it give sufficient space to the cooperation which can exist? Is the apparent concern for the patient merely a smoke-screen for the pursuit of professional privilege by doctors and nurses, or cost cutting by government? Or does this concern underlie improvements in the organisation of health work?

Much of the sociological literature on professions and occupations focuses on the struggle for power and privilege by self-consciously organised workers. There has been a particular interest in the projects of collective mobility of occupations trying to become professions. This chapter will query the narrowness of this focus on the producers and develop the analysis of both their relationship with their clients and with the effectiveness of their mode of organisation of work.

Allies or adversaries?

Doctors and nurses may be considered simultaneously as symbiotically related professions and as competitors. They occupy positions in the medical division of labour in which they need the work of the other to be carried out effectively, so they are mutually dependent workers in the health care team. They are also in a hierarchical relationship in which there is a jockeying for position.

There has long been a tension in nursing as to whether it accepts a clearly subordinate role to medicine or whether it can assert itself as an independent profession with a less unequal status to medicine. This has changed over time from Nightingale's unequivocal declaration of nursing's subordination to medicine, to the Salmon Report's (1968) view that nursing and medicine are independent professions, each with its own internal hierarchy, coming together on a consensual basis.

Medicine's own struggle for autonomy is currently largely in relation to the state, though historically it was against unqualified practitioners. This has affected its relationship with nursing more indirectly than directly. For instance, is nursing to absorb tasks currently performed by overstretched junior doctors that medicine thinks are simple enough for nurses? And who is to manage the budget?

There are different models of the balance between the elements of hierarchy and symbiosis in the relationship between medicine and nursing. In the terms of the Salmon Report (1968) symbiosis takes priority over hierarchy. It represents the epitome of the glorious ideal of the ethical professional. Each profession sees to the achievement of its own standards of professional work. One profession does not, and necessarily cannot, have the expertise to tell the other what to do, since this knowledge resides in one profession only. Hence the relationship between the professions must be one of consensus and mutual respect, if they are to achieve the goal of helping the patient. Each profession has its own hierarchy, and accountability is upward to senior members of the profession. This structure of vertical hierarchies does not easily allow for strong, horizontally organised teams to emerge, since accountability is always upward to the senior of each profession. Teamwork across professions is diminished in significance with this model, and opportunities for innovative change can be missed because of the need to refer back to senior professionals.

> *Registrar (psychiatry)*: One of the tremendous difficulties that you are faced with in a team . . . [is the] fact of one of the members saying 'Well, I'm sorry I can't make a decision about that, I would have to ask my line manager about it.' That's very destructive and I think what you need is some commitment from line management, that they are not going to interfere with the running of that team. Because otherwise you can never make a committed decision within the team, you have always got to be nipping out of the room to ask if I am doing the right thing.

A second model stresses instead the hierarchical relationship between the professions. Here the nurse is the 'handmaiden' to the doctor. The doctors are the lead profession in this model and all other hospital workers are merely auxiliary subordinate occupations. When the doctor directs, the others fulfil their duties. This is based on the notion of the superior knowledge of the doctor as to the best action for the well-being of the sick patient. The contribution of nurses, therapists and carers, particularly but not only in chronic care, is under-estimated in this model.

A third model is somewhere between these two, assuming that there is simultaneously both hierarchy and symbiotic interdependence based on discrete areas of expertise. In this doctors and nurses have different functions, and there is an ambiguity as to the degree to which these functions are 'different but equal', or different and one dominant over the other. The function of the doctor is to diagnose and treat. The function of the nurse is to care for the patient. These can be interpreted as discrete areas of professional responsibility, in which each profession is the best expert of the techniques and knowledge needed. They can also be interpreted as hierarchically related in that, while the doctor diagnoses the patient's illness, the nurse follows the doctor's instructions on the necessary care. The nurse's province of 'caring' is seen as subordinate to that of the doctor's 'diagnosis' and treatment. The functions are both separate and, from a medical viewpoint, for solid, technical, reasons, seen as necessarily hierarchically related. The function that doctors fulfil partially encircles the one that nurses do, restricting the parameters within which nurses do their function. This generates a form of medical dominance over the parameters of nursing and other health occupations. The application of this model generates conflict because the boundaries between the professions are unclear.

All these models exist in the medical sociology literature, the sociology of professions literature, in official reports, in the training undergone by each profession, and among the hospital staff. There is also some historical fluidity between them, sometimes one view takes precedence over the other, sometimes they are in head-on conflict. The history of nursing and of hospitals is the history of the rivalry between these views.

There are, though, elements missing from the debate. There is little formal recognition that different patterns of authority may be appropriate in different health care locations. Medical authority over patient management has a compelling logic when there is acute illness requiring rapid, sophisticated treatment, but the rationale for medical control is far less obvious in the long-term management of disability, or care of frail elderly people. If authority were based entirely on function, and not on status, then it should be possible to identify areas where nurses or, in a wider discussion, therapists controlled the agenda of care. The second point is to question the practicality of dividing the patient into discrete areas of care or treatment, as has already been discussed in Chapter Two.

There are three bodies of literature which illuminate these questions: professionalisation; closure; and labour market segmentation. These will be assessed in the light of our research on the contemporary issues along the boundaries between medicine and nursing, considering both the way the traditional models need to be modified in the light of contemporary developments and whether this debate addresses the most pertinent questions in health work today.

Our study showed complex relations between doctors and nurses which do not fall easily into either the model in which nurses are doctors' handmaids, nor the model of complementary professions. Rather they took different positions at varying times.

The professions

The relations between doctors and nurses are conventionally analysed by sociologists within the framework of the sociology of the professions. Within this literature the focus is on professionalisation as a struggle for occupational advancement at the expense of related occupations and everyone else. At the centre of this debate is power. The detail of the debate is about the diverse ways this power is negotiated. Hence the interprofessional relations between doctors and nurses are frequently understood as ones of a struggle over position and power (Davies, 1980; Gamarnikow, 1978; Mackay, 1989; Stacey, 1988; Witz, 1992).

The debate on professions as a struggle for power superseded an earlier one which analysed professions in terms of their supposed essential characteristics. Writers sought the common traits of professions which made them different from other occupations (Greenwood, 1957; Jamous and Peloille, 1970; Vollmer and Mills, 1966). The distinctive professional traits which were suggested varied on several dimensions. One source of variance was whether the distinctive knowledge base of professions was seen as so theoretical, scientific or complex that it generated an indeterminacy which meant that only the fully trained professional could really be competent in a given sphere, or whether it was merely a set of technical rules to be learnt. A second dimension was the notion of service, which was sometimes seen as being at the heart of professions: specifically, a commitment to altruistic service. A third pointed to the distinctive mode of organisation of the profession: that of self-monitoring, with its own methods of training and assessment of competence. This 'trait' approach has been dismissed as idealist and naive, as taking the professions' self-interested claims about their practices at face value. The statements about altruistic service and specialised knowledge, for instance, have been regarded as a form of self-serving mystification, more rhetoric than reality. The trait approach has been criticised for its failure to concentrate on the more important considerations of power (Freidson, 1970; Johnson, 1972). Despite these criticisms, there is some value in these accounts of key features of professions especially in a concentration on the special relationship between knowledge and forms of occupational control possessed by professions (see, for instance, Larkin, 1983).

One concern of the debate on professionalisation has been the forms of self-governance which are used to pull a profession up the occupational hierarchy. These typically involve forms of closure against would-be practitioners unless they are fully processed by the profession. Themes of occupational hierarchy and occupational closure have been central. Freidson (1970) stresses the significance of the autonomy and control over their work as the basis of professional power, while Johnson (1972) focuses on the relationship of the professional with the client, the control of whom Johnson considers to be the key aspect which distinguishes the power of professions.

The phenomena of autonomy and dominance are sometimes expected to go together, while in others they are distinguished. Distinctions within the notion of autonomy itself may be useful; for instance, between the autonomy of individuals by virtue of their membership of a profession and the autonomy vested in a profession as a corporate body. Autonomy may be separated into economic autonomy, the right to determine levels and forms of remuneration; political autonomy, the right to be considered experts in policy matters related to their field; technical autonomy, the right to determine standards of performance; autonomy over recruitment and training; autonomy in disciplinary practices (Elston, 1991; Freidson, 1970; Larkin, 1983; Ovreteit, 1985; Schultz and Harrison, 1986). National variations in these are also important, and the British concept of 'profession' should not be overextended (Kocka, 1990).

These competing accounts in the social science literature as to what constitutes the key features of a profession reflect the diversity of views of the practitioners themselves. The doctors and nurses in our study had quite different notions of what it was to be a professional. Both groups could justifiably accuse the other of being non-professional; neither showed much sign of realising that this difference existed. This was one of the bases of some of the tensions we observed in everyday working practice. The medical notion of a profession was one where an educated person was able to respond to individual problems in undetermined, innovative yet trustworthy ways. The nursing notion was one of technicality, of pinning down exactly what was to be done and the training and staff needed to do it to agreed standards (cf. Cox, 1992; Jamous and Peloille, 1970; Johnson, 1972).

These dual conceptions of 'indeterminacy' and 'technicality' were frequently echoed in the accounts of the doctors and nurses. Nurses often saw professionalism as being a rule-governed process, intimately tied in with checking and monitoring. Doctors saw a professional as someone who exercised independent judgement. Accounts of disagreements over whether nurses should give IV drugs tied in with this basic difference in approach. Doctors were unable to understand why nursing colleagues put up with rules which stopped them doing work that they were capable of doing. The opposite attitude was expressed by nurses critical of the lack of control and monitoring of junior doctors, or the casualness of doctors when prescribing drugs. However, there has been a paradigm shift in nursing values since the way of authorising nurses through the extended role system of certification was formally abandoned by the UKCC in 1992.

Professions and social structure
Questions have been raised as to the nature of the overall social hierarchy in which professions are located, as well as the position of professions within this. One dimension of the debate here depended upon whether professions were viewed within a Marxist or Weberian conceptualisation of the wider society. The question of the location of the professions in the class structure generated considerable debate, since they were clearly neither simply bourgeois nor proletarian, neither owners of capital nor wage labourers. Their position has been variously characterised as part of the service class (Abercrombie and Urry, 1983); the new middle class (Carchedi, 1977; Johnson, 1977); and the professional–managerial class (Ehrenreich and Ehrenreich, 1977).

Class and capitalism are the wider forms of social structure and inequality which are considered central to the analysis of professions in many of these writings. However, this ignores the patriarchal structuring of society, which is important because of the gendering of the professions, that is, they typically involve men not women. The focus on capitalism has elided the significance of the gender order in the construction of professions (Stacey, 1981), yet professions can only be understood fully in the context of both the patriarchal and capitalist structuring of society (Witz, 1992). This is important, especially when considering the relationship between one profession which is largely male – medicine – and another which is largely female– nursing.

The relationship of professions to the state is a further important theme (Burrage and Torstendahl, 1990; Johnson, 1977; Moran and Wood, 1993; Stacey, 1988; Witz, 1992). Professions usually utilise the state to support their closure projects, to give them legal enforceability. This has been especially important for health professions where medicine was powerfully institutionalised as a result of the 1858 Medical (Registration) Act. Nurses sought a similar state-sponsored form of closure in their campaign for registration between 1888 and 1919, but the Nurse Registration Act which ended that period did not give nurses the same control over their profession that doctors had over theirs (Witz, 1992). The lack of female suffrage during this period was part of the problem of the weaker position of female nurses who had to depend upon male proxies to argue their case in parliament.

The power of the state to interfere in and regulate professions is the other side of the coin. This has come more to the fore in recent years and was forcibly demonstrated in 1993 by new proposals which gave responsibility for the management of normal childbirth to community midwives (Moran and Wood, 1993). Literature on health work is now more likely to discuss the intrusive attention of the state to professional organisation, and to write of tensions between state-paid administrators and managers on the one hand and health professionals on the other (Butler, 1992; Elston, 1991; Harrison et al., 1990; Stacey, 1988; Strong and Robinson, 1990). The work of the general managers introduced in the mid-1980s and their attempts to control health professionals (Harrison et al., 1990; Owens and Glennerster, 1990) is one example among many of the recent tensions between the state and the professions.

The dominant theme of the sociology of the professions is then to assume that the most important part of the professional project is that of gaining and maintaining power and control. Yet, as we have seen from our study, the contemporary relationship of medicine and nursing is more complex than this. Doctors do not always seek the subordination of nurses. Indeed, we have seen instances where doctors have supported the attempts of nurses to improve their position through better training. The complexities of the interactions are better illuminated by the developments in closure theory.

Closure

'Closure' is the process through which an occupation controls entry into itself, and is a practice particularly well developed in professions. Closure involves a set of practices whereby an occupation creates a monopoly over its skills by both controlling entry to training and membership, and by preventing others from practising that trade who have not acquired recognised membership. This monopoly enables the occupation to raise the price of its labour, and is the key to the enhanced rewards and privileges of professions.

The variety of the specific forms of closure used by occupations, including professions, to secure privileged positions form another branch of the literature. Parkin's (1979) analysis of strategies of closure by an occupational group against others was a key development in this literature. 'Exclusionary' closure is used by a powerful group against others less powerful. There are sometimes upward pressures from subordinate groups against the dominant group, which Parkin labels 'usurpationary'.

Parkin's work has been followed by a debate on the best way to conceptualise the diversity of types of closure used by professions and occupations. 'Demarcation' captures the notion of a form of occupational boundary maintenance which is horizontal, between co-equal occupations, rather than downwards in the context of an analysis of labour market segmentation (Kreckel, 1980). Closure can be differentiated according to whether it relates to attempts to control intra-occupational relations or those between an occupation and its neighbours.

'Occupational imperialism' is a concept which captures the way one occupation might exert power over others for its own advantage and is particularly important in the analysis of health work, where medicine has an important role in structuring its neighbouring occupations (Larkin, 1983). For instance, for much of this century medicine has shaped the nature of nursing through such practices as the involvement of consultants in nurse training and in the appointment of ward sisters. Both of these are examples of practices which have been consciously rejected by the nursing profession in the past two decades. Two types of usurpationary pressure can be distinguished: that of those seeking access to the dominant group, and that seeking to change the relations of dominance and subordination altogether (Murphy, 1984).

Gender segregation and closure theory

There is a further angle to professionalisation and closure theory which addresses another fault line in social relations, that of gender. Medicine and nursing are gendered occupations in the sense that they are each composed largely of people of one gender and have structural features related to this gender composition. Both the extent of the gender segregation and the position of women in society are changing: women are now 50 per cent of medical students, although only 15 per cent of consultants. We need to address what significance these gender issues might have for the tension between doctors and nurses.

Most of the theoretical work on closure has been gender blind, though there are important exceptions (Crompton and Sanderson, 1989; Witz, 1992). Witz (1992) integrated a gender analysis into these previously androcentric concepts as well as making distinctions between the exclusionary and demarcationary strategies of dominant group, and the inclusionary and dual closure strategies of subordinate groups. Witz's schema has two dimensions: first, dominant or subordinate group; secondly, exclusionary/inclusionary or demarcatory/dual closure. The second dimension relates to intra-occupational closure as opposed to inter-occupational control. Exclusionary strategies involved forms of closure which operated downwards against other groups (for instance, nursing), while inclusionary strategies were ones by a subordinate group which sought individual access to a dominant occupation (for instance, women's attempts to enter medicine in the nineteenth century). Dual closure strategy involved both attempting to push up against a dominant occupation and to push downwards against others to maintain one's own occupational standing (for instance, nurses seeking state-assisted registration at the turn of the century).

The debates on gender divide over whether gender is conceptualised at a social psychological level (as in the work of Gilligan, 1982) or a structural level (as in the work of Witz, 1992). In the former theory, gender attributes are often seen as a result of socialisation and are deeply rooted in an individual's make up, while in the latter gender is produced as a result of structures including the family, state and labour market. In the former, occupation and behaviour within it are often seen as a matter of choice on the basis of an individual's values. In the latter, the position of the occupation within employment hierarchies is seen as a result of structures of power relations. Here nursing's lowly position as compared to that of doctors is related to the wider position of women in society, the causal links including women's lesser formal political power.

Historical development of medicine and nursing

Professions and occupations cannot be understood simply in terms of the current balance of social relations, but have structures and practices which are rooted in past sets of social relations. The organisational structures of professions have been formed over long periods of time, and there are usually several critical moments at which institutions were formed in a profession's past which affect its current operation. The nature of the historical context at that formative moment, in terms of its forms of class and gender relations, is crucial to understanding how the division of labour between different groups of health workers, including doctors and nurses, was created (Abel-Smith, 1960; Stacey, 1988; Witz, 1992). The development of gender-specific occupations is not an even historical process, but proceeds in sections, with periods of stability and continuity intersected by periods of change and restructuring (Massey, 1984; Walby, 1985, 1986).

This historical dimension is a marked feature of the development of medicine with its rise to pre-eminence in the nineteenth century (e.g. Parry and Parry, 1976). Medicine has often been seen as a leading example of how an occupation can raise itself through occupational closure, state support, and a distinctive body of knowledge. However, today we have accounts which ask about the possible decline of medical dominance in the context of cost-containment policies (e.g. Elston, 1991; Moran and Wood, 1993). Analysis of contemporary concerns which face medicine as a profession have tended to focus on its relation with the state and its managers and administrators.

Nursing has also attempted to professionalise in a variety of ways from the Nightingale model of nurses as pure, obedient, womanly, dutiful, skilled handmaidens of doctors to attempts to obtain state support for a registration scheme which would have provided occupational closure (Gamarnikow, 1978; Stacey, 1988; Witz, 1992). There have been considerable struggles by nursing to become a self-governing, autonomous profession; however, there are varying verdicts on its level of success which has been much less than that of medicine. While Abel-Smith (1960) suggests that it was successful and was part of the emancipation of women, more recent analysts have suggested this professionalisation project was, at best, only partial, because of continuing medical control over key aspects of nursing (Davies, 1980; Stacey, 1988; Witz, 1992). Analysis of contemporary concerns contains some of the same themes as those of medicine, that is, the problematic relation with the state and the new managers (e.g. Owens and Glennerster, 1990).

The nineteenth and very early twentieth centuries were a particularly critical period in the shaping of the institutions regulating contemporary medicine and nursing (Stacey, 1988; Witz, 1992). While Abel-Smith writes a history of nursing as an instalment in the history of the emancipation of women, Stacey considers that, on the contrary: 'By the end of the nineteenth century . . . medical men had established themselves in a powerful position and ensured the subservience of the female occupations of nursing and midwifery' (1988: 96). The foundation of the National Health Service was a further critical historical moment when female nurses were disadvantaged. The failure to involve nurses in the negotiations to set up the NHS was significant and led to problems for nurses thereafter as a result of the way the NHS organisation was structured:

> Plans for what turned out to be the NHS were laid by an administrative and political elite of men working within the medical elite. They were mostly men drawn from the upper middle class. By excluding the nurses not only was the single most numerous body of health-care professionals ignored but one which was composed almost entirely of women and led by them. (Stacey, 1988: 123–4)

Indeed, Bevan consciously rejected the suggestion that nurses should be on the management committees on the grounds that they were not 'experts' (Klein, 1989).

In the nineteenth century occupational closure often involved two separate processes, both direct exclusion of women (ascriptive exclusion) and, simultaneously, closure against the unqualified (often, but not necessarily, women) (Hartmann, 1979; Walby, 1986; Witz, 1992). However, today direct exclusion on ascriptive criteria has largely disappeared, partly as a result of women's citizenship project which has meant the state no longer supports this type of closure project (Witz, 1992). Since women won the vote the state has rarely been mobilised to support patriarchal exclusionary practices. Indeed, it has slowly shifted to a position of opposition to such closure, from the granting of equal pay to women civil servants in the 1950s to the Sex Discrimination Act of 1975. While these are relatively weak pieces of state intervention, in terms of implementing full equality of opportunity for men and women, they are none the less significant in representing a major change in gender policy in the ending of state support for ascriptive closure projects.

The slow working through of the implications of this can be seen in women's increasing entry to the professions. Women take nearly half the undergraduate places at universities, the main gateway to the professions today. Women fill half the training places in medicine, the quotas on women having been removed after the 1975

Sex Discrimination Act. However, women have not reached senior positions in equal numbers, being only 15 per cent of consultants.

Today, the most important aspect of the subordination of women in the health professions is the lowly place accorded to the majority female profession, nursing, which results largely from the circumstances of its historical foundation. This stemmed largely from women's weak position in the public world: without the vote and being dependent upon a few male proxies to push professional closure projects through parliament, a project which was only partly successful because of the power of medicine over nursing which meant that nursing was not self-governing and autonomous.

The implementation of the 1968 Report of the Salmon Committee has sometimes been seen as the high point of the notion that medicine and nursing should be treated as independent and cooperative rather than hierarchically related professions. In 1974, as a result of the Salmon Report, some senior nurse managers were able to participate in planning the health service with doctors and administrators and from that time health teams at local level were run by the consensus of a team in which nurses were represented (although half the committee were doctors) (Stacey, 1988). However, this can also be seen to have been achieved at the expense of exacerbating the internal hierarchy within nursing and in particular benefiting male rather than female nurses. The Salmon Report led to the elongation of the managerial hierarchy in nursing and tended to divide nurse leaders from the rank and file. Rather than simply empowering senior women nurses as managers, the new positions were largely filled by male nurses drawn from the asylum and mental illness areas where they had a significant presence, that is, not by nurses from the higher status teaching hospitals, who were largely female. By 1985 male management of nursing had significantly taken hold and 92 out of 202 (46 per cent) non-regional chief officers were men, although at the more senior level of regional nursing officer there was only one man out of 14. This compares with the fact that among qualified nurses less than 10 per cent were male (Stacey, 1988: 129). The implementation of the Griffiths Report (NHS Management Enquiry, 1983) is widely seen as reducing this high level representation of nurses (Owens and Glennerster, 1990; Stacey, 1988; Strong and Robinson, 1990). The Griffiths reorganisation, which led to the introduction of general managers, took nurses off the key management team. This was fiercely contested and most teams now have a nurse present in some capacity, but nursing representatives at senior managerial levels in hospitals are still very few.

Gender in health work today

The NHS is the largest employer of women in Western Europe, with 79 per cent of its 1,150,816 workforce female (Department of Health, 1988/89). Among nurses and midwives women are 90 per cent of the employees, while among doctors men are 74 per cent (EOC, 1991, citing Department of Health, 1988/89). This generates different patterns and expectations of working. The gendered nature of these occupations is in keeping with those found in the majority of occupations in the West. The women's occupation is paid less, has less training and lower status than that where men are the majority. This necessarily affects the working relationship between the professions and we see that there are a number of instances where the line of tension between doctors and nurses classically represents that between the genders. The clearest example of this is 'tidying up', where (largely female) nurses are generally expected by (largely male) doctors to clean up after them. This expectation crosses over from other gendered areas of life, notably the home, where husbands often expect wives to perform this kind of menial work. Nurses often resent this cross-over of expectations which they consider to be inappropriate in a professional setting.

As well as these gender differences between the occupations there are gender differences within. Men more typically take the higher positions within each profession relative to their numbers, even when they are the minority in the profession, as in nursing. This again is typical of wider gender differences in employment. For instance, among nurses, while it took men eight years on average to reach the grade of nurse manager after initial qualification, it took women on average 18 years. This is only partly linked to child-care related issues, since while women with career breaks took 23 years on average, those who took none still took 15 years (EOC, 1991). A similar pattern emerges among doctors, with women relatively absent at the upper levels: only 1 per 100 consultant general surgeons is a woman. The Report of the Joint Working Party on Women Doctors and their Careers (Department of Health, 1991b), based on an analysis of the progress of doctors over a 23-year period, showed that while women progressed more quickly through their careers up to senior house officer level the trend was reversed at registrar level and beyond, especially at the consultant level (reported in EOC, 1991: 23–4).

This pattern is not unique to doctors and nurses within the NHS but is found in other occupations and in other countries as well. For instance, despite the fact that 79 per cent of the NHS workforce is female, only 17 per cent of its unit general managers and 4 per cent of district and regional general managers are women, while 74 per cent of the ancillary staff and 84 per cent of the administrative and clerical staff are women (EOC, 1991). A glass ceiling for women doctors in America is widely reported (Lorber, 1990).

The EOC report suggests that the absence of consideration of equal opportunities' issues constitutes a major part of the explanation of this situation in the NHS. 'Its employment policies and practices are far from being woman-friendly' (EOC, 1991: 3). The EOC report, based on a survey of all regional and district health authorities in England and Wales and boards in Scotland to which there was an 87 per cent response rate, found that: while 93 per cent of health authorities and boards state that they have an equal opportunities policy, 10 per cent had not put this in writing; 30 per cent had not communicated the policy to their employees; 78 per cent of policies failed to mention sexual harassment; 60 per cent did not have an equal opportunities committee to plan or evaluate progress; 84 per cent did not have a manager whose chief responsibility was equal opportunities; 75 per cent did not monitor the policy and no authority monitored the position of women with children. Indeed, 23 per cent of health authorities and boards still include potentially discriminatory questions on their application forms (EOC, 1991: 4–5). However, there has recently been a specific drive to improve women's position, and each health authority has had to appoint a health authority member to monitor progress.

A major issue is the lack of attention given to the needs of many women who combine paid employment with looking after a household and its implications for the hours of work for which women are available. Women's opportunities for promotion and training are limited; inflexible work patterns prevent women from returning to work after childbirth; part-time work is often only available at the expense of down-grading. While 37 per cent of women in the NHS work part-time, this is 76 per cent of female ancillary staff, 41 per cent of female nurses – 5 per cent of senior grade nurses, 33 per cent of staff nurses, and 37 per cent of enrolled nurses (EOC, 1991: 29) – and only 30 per cent of female doctors. Sixty two per cent of health authorities restrict part-time working to low levels of work; less than 1 per cent of SHOs are working in part-time posts (Department of Health, 1991b: 5). The extraordinarily long hours of junior doctors are incompatible with the demands of parenthood, and the agreement to reduce these to a maximum of 83 then 72 hours is merely a step in the right direction. The EOC notes the irony of consultants having part-time posts in order to facilitate their private work, when part-time work is normally regarded as a less prestigious form of employment (EOC, 1991: 26–32).

There are two ways in which women, as women, have improved their position in health work in addition to equal opportunities policies. First, women have increasingly entered the super-ordinate occupation, medicine. Secondly, they have sought to raise the position of the occupation which has most women, nursing. This is not to say that those who follow these strategies do so self-consciously as women seeking to improve the collective position of women. But rather that as gendered subjects finding their way through a set of gendered social structures, these are the two main routes through which they may seek to obtain the best life chances.

The first instance, that of entry into medicine, follows the battle in the late nineteenth century for women's entry to medical schools and also the 1975 Sex Discrimination Act which made the restrictive quotas on women's entry to these medical schools illegal. Women now form half the entry into undergraduate medical schools, while among the top grade of doctors, the consultants, they are 15 per cent. These are substantial changes in a couple of decades, and still have an in-built dynamic for change as a result of the gender composition of medical students.

The second approach, raising the status of nursing, involves a strategy articulated through a professionalising discourse rather than a gendered one. However, it is an indirectly gendered strategy, even though its practitioners rarely overtly describe it as one, since it leads to the enhancement of the position of a predominantly female occupation. However, this nursing professionalisation strategy appears especially to benefit male nurses, since they take a disproportionately high percentage of the nurse management jobs, thus reducing its overall impact on women health workers.

Gender and professional boundaries

There are two ways in which gender is relevant to interprofessional relations. First, since the occupations are gendered, being disproportionately either male or female, this raises the questions as to whether the conflicts that we saw were also gendered in the sense of drawing on wider social gendered patterns of conduct. A second gender dimension is that of comparing the conduct of different genders within each occupation. Does women's long run socialisation mean that they behave differently from men when confronted with a similar situation? And if so, how? For instance, would women doctors identify with the role of the nurse more than male doctors, or alternatively more strongly assert professional differences to distance themselves from the lower status profession (see Lorber, 1990)? Would male nurses be more assertive in relation to doctors than female nurses and does this generate more tension in their relationship with doctors or, alternatively, does it create the conditions for easier team working with male doctors?

Our study found that the influence of the gender of an individual doctor or nurse on interprofessional conflict was very slight. There were no statistically significant differences in the reporting of conflict or being angry with the other profession at the aggregate level by gender. For each of the conflict-related issues we examined whether the probability of reporting conflict (either explicitly or implicitly as 'being angry') was associated with profession or gender (Table 3.1). Separate analyses for each conflict-related issue using logistical regression was used to analyse the data. While profession was significant on some of the specific issues, as would be logically expected given their categorisation, this was not the case for gender. A near exception was a marginal interaction effect on 'intervention in care of dying patients'.

However, there were a few qualitative comments on other issues which pointed to gender being a significant issue in certain forms of nurse–doctor working. As mentioned in Chapter 2, gender may be an influential factor in the extent to which nurse managers are determined to exclude consultants from any part of the process of appointing ward sisters. The strong impression from interviews was that in the day-to-day work gender is a far more significant factor within professions rather than between them. For instance, at the level of language there is the issue of the use of the terms 'sister' and 'charge nurse', which indicates a male nurse equivalent of a ward sister. Our intention had been to use this ungendered term throughout the text, but we were thwarted by our interviewees, who in four of the five hospitals referred to the person in charge of ward nursing as the ward sister, except in the few situations, mainly on psychiatric wards, where there was a male nurse in charge.

There were some comments about male staff being more assertive, even when they were nurses, although this did not show up in the quantitative data:

Male SHO: There is a difference in the way a male wants to be seen, [males are] more aware of hierarchy.

Male SHO: [Male nurses have] an identity crisis re male doctors in terms of status and power.

Sister: Males are more competitive, try to assert authority more.

Table 3.1   *Conflict-related issues reported by doctors and nurses (by gender)*

	Doctor		Nurse	
	Male	Female	Male	Female
Different opinions regarding treatment	20	2	5	22
Intervention in care of dying patients	5	4	4	10
Lack of respect/courtesy to patients	1	1	1	12
Controlling bad practice	15	5	3	16
Tasks not done	18	9	1	17
Communication failure	7	3	1	14
Bleep	13	7	3	21
Bed allocation, admission, discharge	5	0	2	20
Theatre lists over time	7	1	0	8
Doctor–doctor conflict affecting treatment/care	1	1	2	9
Doctor–nurse manager conflict	16	1	0	1
Low staffing cover/tiredness/stress	15	6	3	10
Personality/attitude to colleagues	11	1	4	22
Won't listen; won't acknowledge colleague's expertise	7	1	2	9
Comments not allocated	6	4	0	8
Total	147	46	31	199

The software package GLIM (Francis et al., 1993) was used for the analysis. A final model was determined by fitting a sequence of models, starting from the interaction model and removing at each stage the least important of the non-significant terms until a final, parsimonious model was obtained where all remaining terms were significant. If an interaction effect was discovered, further statistical modelling was carried out to investigate the interaction in more detail. Statistical testing was carried out using standard likelihood ratio tests between nested models. We are grateful for the assistance of Brian Francis in carrying out this analysis.

There were a number of unprompted comments which suggested that male nurses were treated well:

Female staff nurse: My brother is a male nurse and feels he is treated better by nurses.

Sister: Male nurses . . . are seen as special.

Male charge nurse: As students, males get the cushiest jobs, get let off early, have extended breaks.

Male staff nurse: [Males get] better treatment even from sisters with a reputation for being an old bag.

Male staff nurse: Pampered by other nurses.

These comments suggest that while the male nurse is an outsider, there is an element, at least, of the nursing profession that sees male nurses as treasured outsiders. The contrast in the male/female ratio in hospitals as compared to medical schools was commented on by both male and female doctors. Female medical students are barely half of the students in medical school. Coming into hospital the male doctors may turn their attentions instead to the more numerous female nurses. Some female doctors were amused observers of the different treatment their male colleagues received.

Female HO: Most [female nurses] treat us equally, and treat us as friends equally, and others don't . . . we laugh and joke about it because . . . we are cutting down the potential husband population by being here! It's quite funny for me to sort of stand back slightly and watch, and I do . . . I kid them on about it. . . . I get on with the nurses and it's good, but yeah, they do have it, yes, some of them definitely do have a different attitude to women doctors.

The relative numbers of staff nurses and junior doctors mean that nurses normally set the informal rules for ward relationships at the HO level.

A majority of doctors thought that male doctors had an easier relationship with nurses than did their female colleagues. Female doctors were less likely to make such comments and more likely than male doctors to feel that women doctors had an easier relationship with nursing staff : 38 per cent of the women doctors as compared with 20 per cent of male doctors. There were several comments about flirting which suggested that the sexualisation of the relationship between male doctors and female nurses was regarded by some as improving working relations. This is, of course, not a universally held view. Of doctors, 81 per cent and of nurses, 74 per cent said there was some element of 'flirtyness' in the doctor–nurse relationship (84 per cent response rate).

Gender thus appears highly relevant when looking at the internal hierarchy of each profession, in that men rise to the top more than women, but has only a minor, if any, effect on the nature of the interaction of professionals in conflictual situations. The effect of professional socialisation is more important than gender cultural socialisation in determining professional behaviour in the day-to-day experience of interprofessional working. Female doctors treat nurses in much the same way as male doctors. And male nurses respond in much the same way as female ones. The occupation produces greater homogeneity of conduct for the two genders than would be expected if gender traits were primarily developed in childhood socialisation and were maintained thereafter. Our evidence supports the thesis of the structural determination of gender relations and occupations, rather than the socialisation theories of Gilligan (1982). The bases and forms of conflicts and cooperation are based on the relationship between the occupations rather than the personality traits of their occupants. Nursing and medicine are professions which shape the possibilities of their members, rather than this being primarily a result of the social psychological characteristics they bring with them on entry.

This is not an argument that gender is irrelevant to an understanding of the work of doctors and nurses. Rather it is an argument about the location of the significance of gender. It is when we look at the structural position of doctors and nurses and the formal national negotiations as to their conditions of service, boundaries of duties, and status, prestige and remuneration that gender becomes an indispensable concept for understanding the situation.

The professional projects of medicine and nursing today

The contemporary position of medicine as a profession is still one of the most powerful of all occupations; prestige and remuneration are high, and there is considerable influence over a wide field, including neighbouring occupations, and a wide discursive influence in society, for instance, in the spread of the medical model in social work and the courts. Medicine has become a way of thinking that has broad influence and a commanding authority (see Foucault, 1973; Stacey, 1988). Further, it has deeply rooted institutional bases of power. The basis of medical authority today lies partly in the acquiescence to medical ways of thinking and the pre-eminence of medicine as a scientific mode of thought with amazing practical effects over life and death. Medical discourse permeates widely through society as an authoritative body of knowledge (Foucault, 1973), despite several recent challenges to this superior status. This process of the construction of knowledge operates not only at the level of ideas and beliefs but is firmly rooted in a solid set of social institutions. Medicine is secured through the universities and legitimated by the state. It has highly influential institutions of its own such as the Royal Colleges of Medicine. In the structure of the National Health Service doctors are well represented on the important committees. Crucial elements of the power of the medical profession are its professional autonomy in which it controls its own clinical standards, training and recruitment, collegial based disciplinary procedures and control over the client.

There is a contrary view to that of medicine as the pre-eminent profession which suggests that medicine is losing power, becoming either proletarianised or deprofessionalised. The basis of these arguments is partly technological (there is a decline in the specialness of medical knowledge, for instance, with the introduction of computers) and, more significantly, organisational (for instance, greater scrutiny of costs and procedures by outsiders, either as insurance companies in the US, or as purchasers, or the District Auditor, or Regional Reviews in the UK); finally, there are demands for greater involvement in decision making by patients. While much of the evidence for this downward trend is US based, it should be noted that there are specific ways in which British doctors may be participating in this; for instance, since the foundation of the NHS, they have not had control over remuneration, one conventional dimension of professional power, after they accepted the position of salaried employees of the state. There is a contrast between US and UK doctors in that the former have retained considerable control over their remuneration, but been subject to intrusive monitoring of their clinical practice. By contrast, in the UK they have lost most of their control over remuneration, but significantly maintained control over clinical practice, although these are all subject to qualification and are changing (Elston, 1991; Freidson, 1970; Haug, 1973; McKinlay and Arches, 1985; Stacey, 1988). In our study we have most to say about the dimension of professional control related to clinical and technical autonomy and here significance of the medical control of the client through the 'ownership' of the patient by the consultant was a recurring feature.

Many accounts of medicine tend to treat its practitioners as a homogeneous group. Our study shows that it is very important to differentiate between the different grades of doctors. Junior doctors are not autonomous, nor do they have good working conditions. There is a considerable debate about and effort to improve these conditions, including the attempt to reduce the excessively long hours of junior doctors (Dowling and Barrett, 1991; NHS Management Executive, 1991; SCOPME, 1991, 1992). The pressure on doctors to modify their form of professionalism so that they acquire some greater regard for technical procedures impacts differently on senior and junior doctors. While consultants are being subject to monitoring in medical audit (see Chapter 6), there is a debate as to whether junior doctors should spend more of their training learning routine procedures. For instance, Walker (1991) suggests that 'see one, do one, teach one', is no longer appropriate, given the low levels of competency acquired in this way.

Our study addressed the question of the extent to which there was pressure on the boundary between medicine and nursing today, with either doctors or nurses seeking to redefine this boundary in their favour. Exclusionary downward pressure on nursing by medicine is rarely considered to take an overt form in the UK (unlike the US, see Iglehart, 1987; McKee and Lessof, 1992), though there are indirect processes which link the two in a competitive manner.

The battles which medicine as a profession considers itself to be fighting in contemporary Britain are largely against state interference and against the growth of government orientated managerialism. This is largely a defensive strategy and is discursively represented as a struggle for medical autonomy against government, administrative and managerial interference and a fair budget for health care. These battles have led some writers to reconsider the extent to which medicine is able to maintain its position as an autonomous, elite profession (Elston, 1991; Moran and Wood, 1993).

The introduction of general management in the mid-1980s following the Griffiths Report is widely interpreted as one of the most significant attempts to curtail the power of the profession by managers in the history of the NHS. Medical resistance was enormous and, while in theory unsuccessful in that doctors failed to prevent the introduction of general managers, to a considerable extent it was more successful at the level of everyday decisions than the government had anticipated (Butler, 1992; Harrison et al., 1990; Klein, 1989; Moran and Wood, 1993; Owens and Glennerster, 1990; Stacey, 1988; Strong and Robinson, 1990). These changes are discussed in Chapter 5.

The White Paper *Working for Patients* (Department of Health, 1989a) introduced internal markets, opted out Trusts and medical audit in a continued government initiative to contain and redirect medical expenditure. These measures attempt to place managerial values within medical practice, rather than, as in the earlier attempt, to impose them from outside. Doctors are to measure their own performance and cost, and to compete with each other. Clinical Directorates, usually led by doctors, run their own budgets. Medical audit, by doctors, overviews the cost and performance of individual treatments. Nevertheless, even though doctors are being invited to become their own managers, it is clear that there is a conflict between the values and traditional practice of medicine as a profession and these new modes of governance (Butler, 1992; Department of Health, 1989b; Harrison, et al., 1990; Moran and

Wood, 1993). These changes are discussed in detail in Chapters 5 and 6.

The professionalisation of nursing

Nursing is undergoing a renewed strategy of professionalisation, assisted by the new position of women with formal citizenship rights and access to education. This project has involved major new attempts to develop a stronger scientific and philosophical basis to nursing care, as in 'new nursing' and primary nursing; to improve the level of nurse training and education, as in Project 2000; and a change in the concept and practice of professionalism, as in the recent change in the UKCC code of practice. There is a significant drive to move away from those aspects of the 'Nightingale' tradition that stress the primacy of medical care and to emphasise the holistic concept embedded in her *Notes on Nursing*.

The 'new nursing' seeks to redefine the nurse's role in healing and to claim greater status for it and is represented in a host of new initiatives to boost the profession including the education-led Project 2000 (UKCC, 1986). There has been a significant attempt to build nursing's own body of knowledge with independent forms of training, education and research and a reinvigoration of nursing's claims to have something special to offer the patient in the care that it provides. These have both a practical basis in new ways of working and are underpinned with a renewed philosophical foundation (Kitson, 1993; Robinson et al., 1992; Salvage, 1992; UKCC, 1986).

The 'new nursing' began in the early 1970s. As a movement it drew on the development of new departments of nursing in higher education, the women's movement's challenge to women's subordination in nursing as elsewhere, and consumer demand for reappraisal of the client/expert relationship. A key element is the replacement of a bureaucratic occupational model of nursing for one which is professional. Preparation for the new more demanding role of practitioner was to be provided by higher levels of education. The new nurse practitioner should have greater autonomy. The knowledge base of nursing was to be developed, based on scientifically derived knowledge, but which also involved a movement away from the biomedical model towards a more holistic approach. It draws also on psychotherapy, on humanistic psychology with its emphasis on the discovery of self through honest open relationships with others. The new nursing involves the notion that nursing is a therapy in its own right. The meaningful interaction between nurse and patient can help to mobilise the patient's own resources more effectively in the healing process (Salvage, 1992). There are variations within this movement, for instance, about the extent to which caring should be seen as a therapeutic relationship or as an ethical position (Kitson, 1993).

This model of nursing has been influential in many recent developments in nursing practice, including nursing development units and Project 2000. The Royal College of Nursing has played a key role in developing, disseminating and reproducing it. Three key examples of this are primary nursing, Project 2000 and the change to a more professional code of practice.

Primary nursing has had such a momentum that the influential *Nursing Times* suggested in an editorial in 1991 that it was akin to a 'bandwagon'. In the UK primary nursing was initially developed in the Oxford and Burford Nursing Development Unit (ONDU), and met with hostility from medical staff (Salvage, 1992). As was described in Chapter 2, there is still opposition from some medical staff, but this is not a universal position. Non-nursing managers have also resisted the development of primary nursing, but this has diminished since the concept was given a boost by the demand in the Patient's Charter that each patient should have a 'named nurse'. In practice, this is a concept very different from that of primary nurse, but nurse leaders moved swiftly to capitalise on the opportunity provided (Wright, 1992).

Project 2000 is designed to increase and broaden nurse training, with nurses receiving formal instruction in institutions of higher education, rather than in units attached to hospitals. The curriculum is being made wider to encompass a broader range of subjects and to include more theoretical work. This has involved changing the status of student nurses when they work on the wards from cheap labour to students, with a reduced expectation that they will be just another pair of hands. By early 1993 the transition was well underway with four regions having completed implementation; in the other 10, 65 per cent of pre-registration places had been converted at a cost of £207 million (Friend, 1993; UKCC, 1986).

However, it is unlikely that the nurses' body of professional knowledge will be respected until it is seen to be significant in influencing recovery or promoting health. An accurate estimate of the contribution that nurses make to the treatment and recovery of patients may begin to emerge with the greater focus on outcomes and on medical and nursing audit. Mallett (1991) describes succinctly how effective treatment of acute physical illness depends on the contribution of several health professions, and it is difficult to believe that objective assessment of outcomes will not compel a greater focus on the contribution of nurses and therapists to patient recovery.

Nursing also has to have a different knowledge base in order to claim independence legitimately, hence the significance of nursing's claim to control care, as opposed to treatment. This presents nurses with several dilemmas, including the difficulty of differentiating clearly between care and treatment. In discussing wound management in Chapter 2 the distinction was shown to be far from clear, and the consultant's position as the person with final control over treatment effectively gives the medical profession the authority to pronounce on the limits of 'care'. Nurses also have to distinguish themselves from 'carers' at a time when caring is also establishing itself as a certificated process through the NVQ (national vocational qualification) system. There are clear employment implications.

> Defining what is meant by caring is complex. . . . medical care differs from nursing care; continuous nursing care differs from continuous care. Upon such definitions may depend policies for employment and recruitment. Current debate about what constitutes the nursing task revolves in some measure around definitions; the boundaries between skilled care which can only be performed by qualified nurses, and other forms of care which may be provided by a variety of support or auxiliary staff, are open to negotiation. (Dalley, 1993: 14–15)

Furthermore, for nurses to appropriate caring as entirely their concern suggests an acceptance of the notion that medicine does not have to bother about caring, a position which once stated appears indefensible. Perhaps most surprising, and an issue to which we will return in later chapters, is that nursing has not seized more strongly on a potential claim for a distinctive role through the different location of their responsibilities in the hospital, in that they provide continuous professional care of ill patients where doctors' involvement, though highly significant, is inevitably episodic.

The increase in the skill level of some nurses and the professionalisation project more generally has not been met with unequivocal support by all nurses. Critics contend that only some nurses will be able to follow the professionalisation route, leaving a larger number of nurses as less qualified health care assistants. This is a somewhat narrow viewpoint, in that it ignores the potential of the NVQ system to give open access to the certification process to those who do not possess formal educational qualifications. The introduction of national vocational qualifications for health care assistants offers the prospect of wards in which there are no wholly uncertificated and untrained nursing staff, as opposed to the present mix of qualified and unqualified nurses. So it is possible to envisage a ward with a considerable number of NVQ certificated health care assistants and a much smaller number of registered nurses with clearly defined skill-mix models based on the particular demands of the ward and specialty.

Core issues here are who controls such decisions, and the relative weight given to quality and cost. Carr-Hill et al. (1992) suggest that, as long as general management dominates health care decision making, skill-mix will remain a major issue. It is equally possible that if nursing regained a strong management function it would share the same viewpoint, since attitudes to skill-mix separate out the nurse managers from the 'professionalisers' within nursing. Nurse managers share with general managers a concern to define appropriate skill-mix, while those nurses most strongly identified with the professionalisation strategy want to retain an exclusive right to control the way work is performed.

This is an issue which is actively addressed by the UKCC. For instance, the recent change of official abbreviation for a trained nurse from SEN or SRN to RN is justified on the grounds that it reduces the concentration on the differences between nursing levels, while emphasising the importance of the professional register (UKCC, 1992a). The UKCC is responsible for the registration of the professional nurse but will not be responsible for registering NVQ certificated staff. NVQ staff are likely to join any one of the nursing unions that also look after the interests of registered nurses.

A further issue is over the benefits which accrue to nurses from the new nursing which, it is suggested, are misrepresented as being primarily for the patients. Salvage's critical work is implicitly, though not explicitly, within the framework of the traditional sociology of professions in her interpretation of new nursing. She is rather dubious about claims that new nursing is for the patients' benefit, suggesting that it also benefits nurses: 'Although New Nurses claim to be acting in patients' interests, they are also challenging medical domination and seeking higher status for themselves' (Salvage, 1992: 14). Other studies describe a more positive response among patients, though resistance from doctors. For instance, the Binnie and Titchen three-year study of 'patient centred' care at another Oxford hospital suggested enthusiasm among patients and their relatives (*Guardian*, 19 January 1993: 18–19).

The response of doctors to Project 2000 in our study was hazy, as they were unsure what it would entail. One concern was its impact on the loss of student nurses from the wards, though only a minority of doctors and nurses specifically mentioned this. Doctors typically viewed the skills of nurses as having only a very slight link with formal nurse training. This appears to fit with the perception of many doctors that they themselves learnt to do their work after they qualified and left university. There were some expressions of regret that nurse training would be less ward based and that nurses in the future would have less practical experience and may be less willing to do basic nursing tasks (23 per cent of doctors' comments and 13 per cent of nurses'). There are different motivations from these two groups: most doctors see basic nursing as 'a pig of a job' and cannot envisage any intelligent well-educated person wanting to do basic nursing. By contrast, British nursing tradition has up to now esteemed 'basic' nursing, and these nurse respondents saw the Project 2000 change as a new emphasis that they disliked. But these comments should not be seen as being about responses to up-skilling or down-skilling nurses. It is as if both professions contain people who see Project 2000 as down-skilling nurses, taking away their practical competence, though educating them better at the same time: 'education' being about intellectual understanding and confidence, 'skill' being something different. Some comments about Project 2000 were about a hope that it would help nurses to become more confident and take more responsibility.

> *SHO*: Great if they were more autonomous and took more respons-ibility; they train for four years then ring about giving two panadol.

There is ambivalence as to the implications of initiatives such as Project 2000 which relates to these issues of education, skill and autonomy as the following extract indicates:

> *Medical consultant*: I think nurses can get too much theory, and it's something I'm aware of when I go to specialist units like intensive therapy units or coronary care units. Nurses feel they know best and often there is competition between doctors and nurses which is unhealthy. And I would hate to think that an excessive degree of learning would promote that. I think it possibly will. I think it will possibly induce this element of competition between doctors and nurses and more potential for conflict between what the doctor says is right and what the nurse thinks is right.

> *Interviewer*: Would you welcome clinical nurse specialists such as the stoma nurse, the diabetic nurse?

> *Consultant*: Yes, very much so . . . in fact we've recently done similar in our own unit with a respiratory nurse.

> *Interviewer*: So I'm just trying to make sure that I have got a clear picture of . . . the way you'd like to see development.

> *Consultant*: I think, yes, to have the sort of [ICU type] nurse specialist . . . in great evidence on the wards I think would create more potential for conflict, because of the reason I was saying earlier,

whereas community nurses in this other role can actually supplement very well the work that the doctor can do.

There was general support in our study for more specialist practitioner nurses. Of those who answered the question, 75 per cent approved of these posts and would welcome more. However, there was a minority group who were uneasy about it and saw the nurse practitioner concept as a threat. This varied appreciably by hospital with most unease being felt in Central and College.

SHO: Specialist nurses can be tedious; they think they've got total knowledge; they tell *me* what to do.

Consultant: Can only go so far then they would have to train as a doctor. The worry for doctors is having unqualified people chipping away at the edges; nurses stripping veins . . .

SHO: As long as it doesn't affect our livelihood I'm sure we can come to some compromise.

There was also some unease that nursing would become as specialised as medicine. This was seen as particularly important because nurse staffing shortages mean nurses having to be switched around. Thus we see the continuation of the nurse-as-a-pair-of-hands tradition.

There is a further theme which emphasises the distinction between extending nurses' skills and extending their freedom to make judgements about treatment. Doctors warmly welcome 'their' nurses having more skills, which are seen as helpful, necessary and not threatening to medicine, providing these skills are not threatening to the doctor's sense of being in charge. These attitudes can sometimes also be seen in nurses' responses to specialist nurses, as the following quotes about the same specialist nutrition nurse illustrate:

Medical house officer: HOs hate dealing with [the specialist nutrition nurse]; she hates having to ask HOs to do things she is not allowed to do.

Medical ward sister: The nutrition nurse was pooh-poohed at first; attitudes are changing.

ENT ward sister: [The nutrition sister] changed patient's management without my or consultant's knowledge. She's been booted out of the department, but doesn't know it yet. She will not be invited back.

The nurses' UKCC code of practice was significantly altered in the summer of 1992 to provide a framework for more independent professional judgement to replace the prior system of minute certification. This radically altered the concept of professionalism for nurses. The UKCC, as the regulatory body responsible for the standards of the profession, requires its members to conduct themselves according to rules it lays down. These are issued as a code of practice, which is up-dated from time to time, together with advisory documents which discuss in more detail the implications and meaning of the code.

The second edition of the code of practice, issued in November 1984, was in force while we did our fieldwork. However, in June 1992 the UKCC issued a revised code together with a second broader document on *The Scope of Professional Practice*. Some of the issues between doctors and nurses which we discovered in our fieldwork are the subject of revised attention in the new code and the associated document on professional practice.

In *The Scope of Professional Practice*, issued also in June 1992, the question of 'extended' roles receives new attention.

The Scope and 'Extended Practice' of Nursing

12 The practice of nursing has traditionally been based on the premise that pre-registration education equips the nurse to perform at a certain level and to encompass a particular range of activities. It is also based on the premise that any widening of that range and enhancement of the nurse's practice requires 'official' extension of that role by certification.

13 The Council considers that the terms 'extended' or 'extending' roles which have been associated with this system are no longer suitable since they limit, rather than extend, the parameters of practice. As a result, many practitioners have been prevented from fulfilling their potential for the benefit of patients. The Council also believes that a concentration on 'activities' can detract from the importance of holistic nursing care. The Council has therefore determined the principles set out in paragraphs 8 to 10 inclusive to provide the basis for ensuring that practice remains dynamic and is able readily and appropriately to adjust to meet changing care needs.

14 The reality is that the practice of nursing, and education for that practice, will continue to be shaped by developments in care and treatment, and by other events which influence it. This equally applies to midwifery and health visiting. In order to bring into proper focus the professional responsibility and consequent accountability of individual practitioners, it is the Council's principles for practice rather than certificates for tasks which should form the basis for adjustments to the scope of practice. (UKCC, 1992c: 7–8)

Both the old and new codes clearly state that the interests and well-being of patients and clients should be the first priority. The orientation to the consumer predates the 'reforms' of the NHS and lies at the heart of health professional codes of practice. There is a major change in the principles underlying professional practice in the issue around extended practice in nursing. It states that 'principles for practice' should replace 'certificates for tasks' as the basis of deciding adjustments to nursing practice. It rejects the traditional premises that a nurse's competence is best regulated and evidenced by certificated training. It suggests that the practice of 'extended' or 'extending roles' has led to the limitation of the parameters of practice, and that a holistic concept of nursing care is preferable to one which is based on activities. Developments in care and treatment are considered to be 'the reality' which shapes the practice of nursing. This is a far-reaching change in the principles of professionalism within nursing, and represents a move from a rule-focused approach to one of individual judgement. It moves the nursing sense of professionalism closer to that of the doctors.

While the UKCC makes it clear that the change has been precipitated by the demands produced by reducing junior doctors' hours, our interviews show that many nurses recognise the need for change, and are frustrated by the rigidity of the extended role. Others thought the extended role system satisfactory, and valuable in providing protection against being dumped with responsibility for any task that doctors wanted to discard. The nursing profession is not adopting 'indeterminacy' wholesale. There is a sense of an increasingly confident profession determined to see that medicine and nursing both work to the same rules.

Article 10 of the UKCC code of practice makes it clear that there has to be no shying away from confrontation that is centred round the well-being of patients. A clinical nurse manager justified appropriate confrontation in an article of December 1989 about drug prescribing in the Nursing Board for Scotland Newsletter, *Update*:

> Confronting doctors about badly written prescriptions may cause aggravation but is essential for safe practice. Clause 5 of the Code of Professional Conduct requires that we collaborate and cooperate with other health care professionals, but this does not relegate nurses to a subordinate position. Where Health Boards have no policy for the control of medicines, nurses must insist that this is rectified forthwith. (Farmer, 1989)

There is a question as to whether there will be an equivalent acceptance by the medical profession of the need to move towards a greater element of 'technicality' in the way it trains medical students. Some nurses feel strongly that this is long overdue.

Medicine and the development of nursing

Medicine's response to the development of the nursing profession has historically been mixed, but predominantly there has been a welcome for the improvement in standards of nursing, so long as doctors maintain overall control of the patient. However, in some instances doctors have tried to maintain their right to diagnose and prescribe treatment for their patients against what are sometimes considered undue incursions from nurses. Demarcation issues with nurses are present, though subdued. They take both the form of which profession should do a particular task, often a task which has been changing as a result of new medical technology, and that of the relative significance of the doctor's sphere of diagnosis and treatment and that of the nurse's of caring. Delegation is an enduring issue between doctors and nurses. This is the tendency of doctors to seek to delegate to other health workers, including nurses, tasks which have become simple or onerous. The practice of delegation means that the control of the task remains with the doctor, rather than becoming part of the sphere of control of the nurse. This has involved a series of tightly negotiated local agreements whereby nurses could be specially trained to do specific tasks, known as the extended nursing role. Within a closure perspective this is a renegotiation of the demarcation with medicine. It may involve 'dumping' on nursing. However, alongside 'dumping' may exist a desire for nurses to become more skilled, the better to do their job and to assist doctors in theirs.

Indeed, this desire that nurses should become more professional and exercise more responsibility was a recurring theme in our interviews. This is not the response of a defensive profession under threat from a neighbouring professional rival. We found that doctors were uneasy at the theoretical idea of nurses taking on technical responsibilities that encroached on to medical territory, but in practice they encouraged this with 'their' nurses on 'their' ward or department. Medical staff want to have highly qualified and competent nurses, so long as they do not overtly challenge the domain of the consultant. There were several examples of medical support for programmes to extend nursing skills, especially in ICU and A&E departments, and the appointment of specialist stoma and diabetic nurses.

In ICU, nurses are very highly trained and often perform procedures and use machinery confidently that consultants from other departments may not be able to manage. ICU nurses estimate blood gas levels, decide on appropriate levels of sedation within quite wide parameters set by the doctors, manage intravenous fluid administration, and generally have technical responsibilities beyond what most non-ICU doctors could manage, and are totally supported by their consultants in this role. If doctors were to be threatened by the rising skill level of nurses then ICU departments should have contained leading examples of this. In fact, the consultants here were proud of the skill of their nurses, and full of praise for their professionalism and ability. Somehow these skills were not perceived to stray onto any territory that the doctors wished to keep for themselves.

A&E departments often now have a 'triage' system which means that the triage nurse assesses the patient's condition when he or she arrives in A&E, and decides who should be a priority case. In some hospitals the system has moved on to having nurse practitioners who see to minor injuries. It is difficult to define an exact point where 'assessment' and 'diagnosis' differ, but it is consistently stated by both doctors and nurses that diagnosis is a doctor's responsibility. A dispassionate study of some of these changes would suggest that nurses have taken on responsibility for 'diagnosing' minor conditions. But providing this is not called diagnosis and is done with the approval of medical colleagues, doctors are not threatened. The extension of a nurse's role in this way is acceptable. This might be considered 'flexible' working.

There are some nurses now trained to assist in vein stripping operations, associated with the Radcliffe at Oxford, a quite overt movement of nurses into the surgical team. This arouses disquiet among some nurses, as well as some doctors. Nurses see this as not being nursing, and see such nurses as having been manipulated into a medical and managerial agenda that supports the view that nurses are a pool of cheaper substitutes for doctors, which is a rejection of 'real' nursing. This development has not been blocked by doctors, but was viewed as a threat to medical power by several doctors interviewed.

There were a few exceptions to the medical acceptance of increasing nursing skills and their arenas of action, but they were more to do with nurses' attempts to change the mode of ward organisation than technical skills. Sources of tension included the introduction of primary nursing, which changed the way a consultant would have to relate to nurses; the question of whether consultants had a right to be involved in the appointment of a ward sister, which they had recently lost; and the loss of consultant input into nurse training consequent upon the move of much training out of the hospital into the colleges.

Community nursing was outside our area of empirical research, but it is worth noting a very significant change in the new right of community nurses to prescribe a limited range of drugs. This has been formally enacted through parliament. The significance of this shifting boundary between doctors and nurses in the community is likely to grow because of the challenge of how to provide care for people with chronic conditions satisfactorily, cost effectively and in line with patients' wishes – and that often has to mean at home. There is a widespread movement towards de-hospitalisation, with far more emphasis on day surgery and day treatment, on rapid discharge, and on hospital-at-home patterns of care. Recent announcements indicate that this process is likely to accelerate, with an associated programme of hospital closure. (*Guardian* 29 September 1993). All of this is likely to challenge the boundaries of nurse–doctor territory, because it will be impossible to provide the same team of medical staff in the community as in hospital, so that there will inevitably be some movement of responsibility for particular tasks that in hospital are undertaken by the most junior doctor. GP practice nurses routinely take blood samples, and some do cervical smear tests, both tasks that would not necessarily be considered nursing duties in hospital.

In summary, consultants are supportive of nurses in their own specialty expanding into territory that would have been considered exclusively a medical domain only a short time ago, but are threatened by generalised statements about nurses becoming 'practitioners', or any hint that nurses diagnose or prescribe. Newly qualified doctors may resent nursing's claims, but if so, it is for reasons much more closely linked to their own uncertain status. Dominant attitudes are set by the consultants.

There is a dilemma for nursing. Medicine sets the level of the upper ceiling, so if they go up-market to professionalise they move into a medical area. If they try to move up to a managerial role they meet a male-dominated world that does not welcome them, and their own safe career ladder of nurse management is being broken down. Nurses are under pressure from two further directions: sideways from the development of therapists, such as occupational therapists, physiotherapists and social workers; and from below by carers – care assistants in the community and health support workers in hospitals.

Nurses have met more resistance to their professionalisation project from those who run the hospitals than from doctors. This is the case not only today, but historically (Witz, 1992). A concern of hospital administrators and managers is that of keeping down the cost of nursing. A further limitation has been the lack of cohesion in nursing ranks, where some fear increased divisions in nursing separating a small elite from a larger less skilled body. Indeed, in tussles with managers, notably over the nurse grading exercise, where nurses were placed on a new grading structure, with many resulting grievances from nurses over their location, doctors have often allied themselves with nurses. This is partly out of loyalty which comes from being part of the ward team, and partly from a sense of shared perspective with a related medical profession as opposed to managers.

Indeed, medicine's relations with nursing are often a by-product of their larger struggle with the state (Robinson, 1992). Struggles over budgets have important effects for nurses on whom most of the budget is spent. Junior doctors are widely regarded as currently overburdened and working hours which are too long. As part of an agreed policy to reduce the excessive hours of junior doctors in hospitals there has been a search for ways of reducing their workload: either by obtaining more money for more doctors, or by handing over some of their work to nurses, clerical staff and technicians. This has implications for medicine's relations with nursing.

The Standing Committee on Postgraduate Medical Education (SCOPME, 1991) report, following on from the NHS Management Executive report *Junior Doctors: the New Deal* (1991), suggested that junior doctors be relieved of some tasks, some of which were to go to nurses, and some to clerks and porters. The tasks which were recommended to go to nurses were: simple suturing; administration of intravenous drugs; and 'topping up' of epidurals. The tasks which were recommended to go to technical, clerical and administrative staff were: locating empty beds; delivering requests and obtaining results of laboratory tests; portering duties; routine blood taking; and filing results in case notes. The tasks which were to go to nursing were the ones which were considered to be simple enough tasks for nurses to do. These themes are reflected in numerous articles in the *British Medical Journal* on the plight of junior doctors and suggestions for which work could be passed to others. For instance, the increased workload on IVs could be done by nurses or junior doctors on shifts according to Denton et al. (1991) and by nurses, following US practice, according to Fisher (1991). In terms of closure theory this might be interpreted as the dominant occupation attempting to re-draw the demarcation line with the less powerful occupation by dumping simple tasks on the latter. It is a strategy which would enhance the position of medicine in the occupational hierarchy.

Conclusion

Theories of professions and occupational closure which focus on a struggle for power against adjacent occupations are not adequate for an analysis of the contemporary interprofessional relations of medicine and nursing. The two professions are significantly complementary as well as competitive. There are shifting patterns of alliances which at times see the doctor and nurse cooperating against intrusions from either senior nursing staff or other consultants; between doctors and nurses in opposition to the programmes of general managers; and between general managers and nurses; and between general managers and doctors.

There are tensions between the professions. The nurses have a current project of developing their profession which might be considered to be competitive to that of doctors. These occur first where nurses try to resist a handmaid role, as for instance in the example of tidying up and, secondly, where there is an attempt to give greater priority to nursing's concern with care than with doctors' concern with treatment, as in the examples of tension around respect for the patient and over care for the dying. However, while such issues generate some tensions, they are not the major source of tension between doctors and nurses. On more important issues, such as nurses' increasing levels of skill and training, doctors were largely supportive and did not see this as a threat to themselves, rather an aid. There were some areas where doctors appeared to be more than willing to relinquish a previously medical task to nurses, such as IVs, which could be interpreted as the doctors dumping less prestigious work on nurses. Indeed, we see as much tension from doctors trying to get nurses to do more, and nurses' resistance to taking on extra work, than from doctors resisting an extension of the role of nursing. There were some difficulties which originated in the widely divergent conceptions of professionalism held by nurses and doctors, but this was typically of a form which wished for greater rather than lesser professionalism, and for a form of professionalism closer to that of their own. However, there were limits to this welcome for nurses improving their position. When nurses improved skills which the doctors could direct, they were pleased. But when nurses developed skills which were outside of the doctors' control, the doctors were less pleased.

The doctors who were most vociferous in challenging nurses' skills were the most junior doctors. The development of nursing skills is not a threat to consultants and the more senior registrars, but does produce frequent tussles over authority with house officers and SHOs. At times nurses collude with consultants in order to control the decision making of junior medical staff.

Doctors in the NHS hospitals we surveyed generally did not feel threatened by the nurses' professionalisation project. The upskilling and increased training of nurses was generally within the range of behaviours they wished for in nurses. Better skilled nurses were an asset not a threat. The model of competitive professions is not the most appropriate one with which to understand the tensions in interprofessional working, although some examples of this could be found. The tensions are as likely to arise from the fragmentation of the doctor–nurse team under pressure. It is to examples of this that we turn in the next chapter.

4

Fragmented and Functioning Teams

In the UK, the 1980s saw the beginning of an unprecedented drive to improve the efficiency of the National Health Service. Continual downward pressure on costs has subsequently been exerted through mechanisms such as cost improvement programme targets, and an obligation on managers to achieve a balanced budget.

There is a basic question: what form of management process is the NHS using in the 1990s to produce 'efficiency'? From 1985 the NHS encouraged efficiency through a general management system. Efficiency was, and is, measured by the 'output' of the hospital as an institution, as shown by increased throughput of patients and high bed occupancy rates. This is entirely in keeping with the concentration on mass production associated with older styles of centralised management control, which we refer to as Taylorism. When the output of the hospital as a whole is the primary focus, the ward-based teams of doctors and nurses are not, in themselves, a matter for concern.

With 'new wave' management, the devolution of decision making to semi-autonomous teams is, in contrast, seen as an issue of fundamental and central importance. Efficiency is concerned with the responsiveness of the team to the patient, and successful outcome has to be seen to relate to individual patient, or 'customer', satisfaction as well as hospital output. The documents that emerge when NHS hospitals apply for Trust status are written in language that reflects this kind of management thinking.

Quite apart from the direction of policy, the nature of hospital organisation is such that nurses and doctors do not always form cohesive ward teams. Within a Taylorist tradition, this is not a very significant matter. Consultants admit and discharge patients, so they control turnover, and they also determine many costs by the decisions they make. So if the focus of management concern is closely linked to turnover and costs, consultants are the only professional staff group whose decisions greatly matter. When there is a determination to encourage the devolution of responsibility to the staff who deliver care and treatment different values emerge. It is against this background that we examine how the drives for efficiency combine with the nature of medical and nursing organisation in hospital to influence the work of medical and nursing staff.

Medical and nursing staff are two groups of professionals who are concerned with the care and treatment of the same group of patients, but who operate in different geographical locations around the hospital, and arrange the provision of 24 hour care in strikingly different ways. Doctors move round the hospital from wards to outpatient clinics, to the accident and emergency department, to the path lab, to theatres sometimes, and often to a different hospital. Night time and weekend cover is provided by on-site and on-call house officers and SHOs, backed up by more senior medical staff, on-call, but off-site. Hence we see the most junior doctors on call for 70–80 hours, twice as many hours a week as most people consider an ordinary working week, and sometimes more. Doctors will work across several wards, wherever patients in their specialism are located.

By contrast, the majority of nurses stay on one ward or department, and the patterns of employment for nurses are much more tidy and bureaucratic than they are for doctors. Nurses work shifts and have timed meal and coffee breaks. The thirty seven and a half hour week that nursing staff officially work is usually spread over five days, but intensive three day systems are preferred by some staff, and on some wards there are internal rotas to cover night duty. Nursing employment contracts are based on the idea that staff go off duty when they have worked their time, not when the work is 'done', and though, in practice, nurses frequently work over their allotted time, the timed shift is the basic employment model. Most nurses are ward based and are accountable for the care of the patients on their ward. Staff are moved for a few hours, or for the duration of a shift if there is extra demand on a different ward. Nurse managers control the distribution of nursing staff within a specialty.

The doctor–nurse ward team exists, but it is not a group of staff routinely working together, rather one that meets regularly, but often briefly and in passing. Medical and nursing staff orbit along different trajectories, nurses in one location but through a 24 hour shift system, doctors around the physical geography of a hospital or group of hospitals. This difference we refer to as 'the time–space geography' of medicine and nursing. It presents practical difficulties in maintaining effective information exchanges, and creates different patient care priorities.

Such differences can normally be accommodated without difficulty, but the separate agendas of medicine and nursing create tensions when there is continual strain on resources, particularly on staffing levels. For the past decade funding pressure has been such that attempts are continually made to maintain traditional service provision with less relative spending, while new patterns of staffing mix and staffing provision are simultaneously introduced in an attempt to contain costs. There is no sense that the pattern of change is slowing, and the need to find ways of reducing the unacceptable number of hours worked by junior doctors is adding another element of change (Audit Commission, 1991; Butler, 1992; Harrison et al., 1992).

The working patterns of doctors and nurses in hospitals have always differed, and there has been long experience of working under pressure. It is the change in the way hospitals are organised that has added a different kind of pressure on staff. Increased throughput of patients and tighter cost and budgetary controls have been introduced in order to meet demands for increased efficiency. There has been increased surveillance of working practices, increased managerial intervention and increased managerialism within the professions. In interviews with ward staff we saw how policies to improve bed occupancy rates, and policies to control ward budgets and increase throughput were interacting to fragment the sense of a coherent, ward-based, nurse–doctor team. When the commonality of the nurse–doctor ward team is weakened some conflicts become persistent. This pattern emerged with clarity in some accounts of disputes relating to admissions, and bed alloca-tion, and also in theatre use and on high turnover wards. It was, though, also noticeable that the extent to which staff saw themselves as working well as a team varied between hospitals, and that within each hospital particular specialties, though not always the same ones, reported more frequently that there was consistently good teamworking between the two professions.

The probability of teamwork

Interviews were conducted in five hospitals: Greenfield, College, City, Central and County. In interviews with medical and nursing staff respondents were asked if they felt that doctors and nurses 'worked as a team'. Only 12 per cent felt that this never happened; 55 per cent reported that it routinely happened; and 33 per cent said it occurred sometimes, on some wards. Table A1 in the Appendix (see p. 183) shows the distribution for both nurses and doctors from each hospital and for each specialty. The information gained from this question was of considerable value in comparing responses from similar specialties in different hospitals, but there were difficulties in the data. One problem was that doctors who worked in more than one hospital did not always distinguish between them. Their answers were also more likely to be referring to a group of wards, rather than one ward, which was the focus of nurses' attention. Further, the question left it to respondents to distinguish between the ward-based medical staff and visiting doctors coming in to see patients. The latter is doubtless a factor affecting responses from intensive care, and from ENT.

We investigated using logistical regression whether the probability of responding that staff 'worked as a team' varied according to the profession of the respondent, the specialty, and the hospital. We have called this the 'probability of teamwork'. The results from the statistical modelling indicated that the probability of teamwork depended to a varying extent on these three factors, and that, moreover, the specialties that have a high probability of teamwork are different for nurses and doctors. The interaction between speciality and profession is mainly explained by different professional reactions to general medical and surgical departments. Doctors have high probabilities for medicine and psychiatry, while nurses have high probabilities for surgery, theatre and A&E. There was no evidence of an interaction between profession and hospital, or between hospital and specialty.

The hospital effect was marked, with Greenfield giving the highest probability of teamwork, and College staff the lowest probability. The full ranking is shown in Table 4.1. A similar table

Table 4.1   *Working as a team: analysis by hospital (doctors and nurses)*

		%
Greenfield	41/56	73
Central	30/48	63
City	23/42	55
County	20/45	44
College	22/56	39
Total	136/247	55

(Table 4.2) was constructed to give the distribution of people who reported that there had been no recent conflict on the ward. This was also analysed using logistical regression, the result showing no evidence of any effect of speciality or profession. The only effect found was a strong hospital effect, with Greenfield having the highest probability of no recent conflict and Central the lowest.

The ordering of the hospitals is similar in both tables, with the

Table 4.2   *No recent conflict: analysis by hospital (doctors and nurses)*

		%
Greenfield	29/56	73
City	19/50	38
County	15/50	30
College	15/55	27
Central	9/49	18
Total	87/260	33

exception of Central, which falls from second to fifth place, suggesting that conflict is no barrier to teamwork. This discrepancy between 'good teamworking' and 'no conflict' makes it clear that differences of opinion can be accommodated within effective teams. The contrasts that emerge between Greenfield and College are striking, and are further discussed later in this chapter, but it is first necessary to explore how hospital pressure, and the geography of hospital care, affects ward teamwork.

Ward teams and conflicts

In Chapter 2 we described some accounts of nurse–doctor conflict. Table 2.1 quantified all accounts of nurse–doctor conflict as reported by ward staff. The second category related to problems of time–space geography, especially when under pressure of resource scarcity. For ease of reference these are repeated in Table 4.3. They were cited in a significant number of instances of conflict, only slightly less often than those generated by professional boundaries.

Table 4.3   *Conflict issues relating to time–space geography under pressure*

	Doctor	Nurse	Total
Bleep	20	24	44
Low staffing cover/tiredness/stress	21	13	34
Bed allocation, admission, discharge	5	22	27
Communication failure	10	15	25
Theatre lists over time	8	8	16
Total	64	82	146

Of these items the more intense conflict occurs when staff are tired, and working with staffing levels that they perceive as inadequate. Theatre lists are a particular case of staffing pressure. These two categories, low staffing cover and theatre lists, are discussed first, then bed allocation, bleeps, and communication failure.

Low staffing cover
Budgetary pressures are most keenly felt over the issue of nurse and theatre staffing levels. Various formulas are used to give an apparently objective assessment of the staffing levels required, but until recently none of these was able to command the support of both professional and management staff. Nurse staffing costs are the largest single item of hospital budgets, so when there is pressure on finance, and no consensus, nurse staffing levels are a focus of controversy.

Admissions cause conflicts between medical and nursing staff, particularly when nurse staffing cover is seen by nursing staff, and often by medical staff, to be unacceptably low. While doctors and nurses may both accept that nurse staffing is inadequate, their response is often markedly different.

> *Registrar*: One of the theatre sisters was under a lot of stress because of staff shortages and she was more or less wanting us to cut down on our patient admissions to enable them to cope . . . you could see the frustration in her face, she just felt like packing it up and going away . . . if I challenge her she will deny that she's asking me to do so, because she knows it is not correct . . . I found it unacceptable. If she has a staffing problem she should talk to management to provide staff . . . but management cannot provide staff so they shuffle staff from one department to another to try and make up, but it doesn't . . . She expects understanding from us, but at the same time, we want to make sure that our waiting list is cut down.

> *Consultant*: It really was just the duration of pressure on work load . . . when this goes on for two or more months, and patients begin in [nurses'] eyes definitely to suffer because of it, then they begin to get very upset . . . having tried to get extra staff through their own nursing side, and been unsuccessful, then they try to put pressure on medical staff not to admit so many patients. Medical staff say well, we can't do that, and that's when the arguments begin. Then each patient that's admitted is being scrutinised to see if it is really a necessary admission and if there is the slightest doubt whether it is necessary then it creates disharmony. The tension is primarily due to lack of funding, I would say that is the main cause, and I have noticed it increasingly over the last five years. The problems are not of actual workload, it is of being asked to do more and more with fewer and fewer resources and staffing.

When doctors see that their wards are inadequately staffed criticism is often directed at nurse managers, since this is the group with the unenviable responsibility for ensuring that all the wards in their area are adequately staffed with the right mix of nurses at different grades. Nurse managers are caught in the quintessential health care trap; responsibility for producing an expensive resource, and responsibility for balancing their budget. At the time of our interviews, a few nurse managers were still able to overspend. Most were not so fortunate. Maintaining an adequate staffing level over all the wards meant a very careful balancing act, and one that received scant sympathy from consultants solely concerned with one or two of those wards, particularly if inadequate nurse staffing meant that patient admissions had to be reduced.

Senior nurses, both sisters and nurse managers, are aware that nurses like to be helpful, and that they can be persuaded to take on extra duties. Once nurses carry out a task a few times it becomes expected that others will do the same. When staffing levels are tightly defined, and it is difficult, sometimes impossible, to provide good quality nursing care, senior nursing staff see a need to be constantly vigilant that doctors do not transfer extra work on to nurses. Tightly defined staffing levels produce tightly defined task boundaries as nursing staff dig in their heels to resist being overwhelmed with responsibilities. The responsive, flexible, autonomous, multi-disciplinary team dreamed of in the aspirations of 'new wave' managers becomes a wary, inflexible group of staff defensively marking out the limitations of their responsibilities.

> *Sister*: We're not staffed to look after the out-patients but they often want us to take dressings off, stitches out, or they say 'you can give me five minutes can't you', and I say 'no that's your remit not mine', and they get . . . huffy about it, but I mean we're actually employed for the in-patients. It's tried on with different staff nurses . . . it's just got silly in that they know we can't do this, we just haven't got enough staff.

To a junior doctor decisions often appear arbitrary and petty.

> *House officer*: This morning, I had to take out sub-cutaneous pacing wire . . . which is simple you just cut some stitches and pull . . . there's very little risk that anything can happen . . . And the consultant asked the staff nurse on the ward round to do it . . . she agreed . . . and I get paged at 4.30 in the afternoon to say that they're not going to do it any longer and it's your job.

Stress and tiredness

Nursing is often physically demanding, heavy work. The same tasks have to be repeatedly performed, and some of them are unpleasant.

Nurses know that their work is sometimes denigrated as 'shovelling shit'. They see themselves and their work devalued, and at times describe themselves in these terms. Job satisfaction comes from seeing patients make some progress, or being able to relate to the person, rather than concentrating on completing tasks. Low staffing levels, or very high turnover, can mean that care has to be rushed and patients have to be processed through a cycle of tasks. At the end of the shift there is little sense of having completed anything worthwhile. The combination of low morale and physical tiredness leads to a desire to simply get through the work and go off duty. A doctor who recognises the level of work pressure on nursing staff and comments sympathetically earns considerable respect.

This is less likely to happen when the doctor is also tired. Several of the areas of tension between doctors and nurses have been significantly exacerbated by the deterioration of the position of junior doctors over the past couple of decades. The intensity of the work and the turnover has increased but the hours have not changed. Consultants' experience of their own period as house officers was of an easier life than that currently experienced by junior doctors. Excessive hours of work, sleep deprivation and several nights with a limited range of meals re-heated in the dining room microwave do little to enhance cooperative teamworking. Several accounts of disagreement relate to this problem of the long hours of junior doctors: bleeps, tidying up, IVs are all areas where the overwork of the junior doctors places stress on the relationship with nursing staff.

Another factor which caused much resentment among junior doctors was the fact that the nurses they regularly worked with often showed no understanding of the long hours they work on their on-call weekends. Junior doctors feel justified if they are short-tempered at the end of a long weekend on call and have little respect for nursing colleagues who do not make allowance for the level of exhaustion they experience. To be criticised for being moody or unfriendly is intolerable. This doctor's account is similar to many comments from junior doctors.

> SHO: A particular weekend [when] I'd been called to see a patient at seven o'clock in the morning, I'd only got four hours sleep in the last 80 . . . and the sister had called me out and said I was not exactly cheerful . . . which just . . . I just blew my top!

Listening to several accounts like this, and to equivalent descriptions from nursing staff about medical failure to appreciate their workload, compels a realisation that neither profession adequately prepares its staff to be effective members of a multi-disciplinary team with colleagues who have strikingly different working patterns.

Much depends on the innate capacity of individuals to recognise when colleagues are under extra work pressure. The more wards that doctors have to visit, the less likely it is that they will be working with nursing colleagues with whom there is some mutual understanding of fluctuating patterns of work stress.

The different patterns of shifts, rotas and breaks between doctors and nurses generated resentment from doctors when there was no nurse to assist them, but where they could see nurses were going off the ward. Nurses work shifts and have strictly timetabled meal and coffee breaks. This attention to the clock is considered by doctors to be unprofessional; doctors do not have timetabled breaks and are often on call rather than off duty. Hence doctors and nurses have different patterns of availability and attitude to the balance of work and rest time.

However, this difference represents not only different notions of what is professional, but also differences in the gender of the two professions in that one typically has a partner to cook his dinner while the other is likely to have a family demanding one; one is likely to have a partner or paid help to see to children, while the other has to do this herself. It will be interesting to see if doctors' attitudes change if they start to work shifts, as some solutions to the crisis in junior doctors' hours have recommended.

Theatre lists over time
Operating theatres are booked to surgeons at specific times of the week, with emergency theatre facilities available at other times. If a particular surgeon's operating list goes over the allotted time then it will demand adjustments to the work pattern of several groups of staff: anaesthetists, theatre nurses, any surgeon wanting emergency operating time, recovery room nurses, operating department assistants. It is quite possible to manage extra demands on theatre time if the theatre budget can pay for extra staff, but if this is not possible then the inherent conflict between demand for professional time and willingness to work extra hours cannot easily be settled.

At each hospital staff described tensions between surgeons and anaesthetists over the use of theatre time, but the frequency with which lists went over time varied significantly between hospitals.

> *Senior registrar*: Surgeons are, by nature, immensely optimistic people, quite convinced that they can do something when they can't . . . I mean commonly we have more patients listed for surgery, than could realistically be done . . . every day, things are rearranged, and we do cases at other hours if there are problems, even sometimes cases off lists are done on a Saturday if there's been unwarranted problems.

Theatre sister: The only thing that I would say is a grouse is if the surgeons run over time, but that happens very, very seldom in this hospital.

If lists go over time disagreements about whether to continue the list may be between surgeons and anaesthetists, or anaesthetists and surgeons may be agreed and the debate is over the need to use on-call emergency theatre nursing staff, or to have the existing nursing staff work extra hours. Anaesthetists programme their time tightly and need to have fairly precise cut-off points. Surgeons claim that their own attitude is the correct professional one, they don't have a cut-off point: 'If the work is there to be done we do it.' In staffing theatres, anaesthetists have to be managers of an expensive facility spread over many sites, while surgeons are concerned with the particular patients they want to treat at that time. Some disagreement is inevitable.

If it is necessary to ask nursing staff to work extra, or bring in on-call staff, there are staffing costs that have to be met from the theatre nurse staffing budget.

Sister: I go to [the nurse manager] and say that this is happening all the time, the nurses are having to do over-time, but if he is worried about his budget then he doesn't want over-time to be done.

An alternative to paying for extra hours is to offer nursing staff extra time off, but this can only be a short-term solution. The demands on staffing time mean that nurses cannot easily be given extra hours off out of their contracted hours, and when nurses build up the number of hours they are due, and do not get any extra time off, they begin to resist calls to work extra hours. Surgeons who work unspecified hours see the nursing staff's insistence on regular hours as a dereliction of duty. Anaesthetists work closely with theatre nursing staff, and may be more aware of outside pressures on nurses. Theatre Users Committees attempt to sort out recurrent problems of theatre use, but in some hospitals disagreements were commonplace.

Bed allocation, admission, discharge

Finding a bed for a patient can be a source of problems, with doctors seeking to admit a patient and nurses protesting that the nursing staff are over-stretched or not expert in the nursing care of patients requiring admission. A doctor may be trying to find a bed for a newly admitted emergency patient waiting in the A&E department, while nurses are trying to hold on to a couple of empty beds to make sure that the waiting list patients booked for admission in the morning will not have to be deferred. Hospital procedures vary. Some hospitals give overt responsibility for this task to doctors, or to nurse managers. Unit managers are also involved in supplying information updates and deciding general policy.

> *Unit manager:* We try very clearly to make it a medical responsibility to find the beds . . . they're the ones that can create the beds by identifying those patients that can move out to another hospital or be discharged . . . Sometimes the pressure on beds has been such that the doctors do a ward round in the morning, we tell them in the afternoon if we don't think there are enough beds to take them overnight, so the doctors do another ward round in the afternoon to see if any patients have progressed enough to go home . . . we know we need roughly twelve empty beds [for emergencies] at this hospital at night. Some of the doctors would love to say to the nurse managers, well you find a bed for this patient, but we try to discourage that.

Sometimes a major part of the responsibility for finding a bed falls on the shoulders of the house officer, or junior doctor who is admitting in casualty. It is an area where the differing loyalties of the two professional groups may be starkly revealed. The junior doctor urgently needs to find a bed for the patient in casualty, and the loyalty is to that patient. The nurse in charge of the ward is aware of the needs of the two or three dozen people on the ward, may be conscious of the lack of skills needed to nurse the potential new admission adequately, and has a primary loyalty to the patients they see and know on the ward. A new admission of a seriously ill patient may in practice quite markedly diminish the quality of care that the nursing staff can give to existing patients. While there is always an acceptance of the ethical duty to admit ill patients, it is legitimate to argue that the patient's needs would be better met by admission to a different ward or unit which theoretically could offer more skilled care, or may be considered to be under less pressure.

It has to be assumed that many emergency admissions run smoothly, but we listened to a sufficient number of accounts of difficulties to appreciate the tensions that can arise with emergency admissions to already very busy wards. There is also some tension over whether to accept the clinical judgement of a house officer. It is the house officer who is more likely to be directed that a patient requires specialist care.

In the following account a house officer was faced with conflicting pressures: from the casualty unit to move the patient to a ward; from a coronary care unit already full; from his own clinical doubt about whether it was necessary to monitor the patient's heart beat; and from a staff nurse aware that nurses could not take on the extra and unfamiliar responsibility of cardiac monitoring. The fact that inter-personal relations were excellent was irrelevant on this occasion.

> *House officer*: The patient was needing a cardiac monitor, and there's no monitor on this ward, if [the patient] needs to be monitored they go to cardiac care, and recovery room staff were pushing me to clear the patient out of there. I wasn't prepared to get the patient out, 'cause I thought he needed a rest, you know . . . I rang the senior registrar in a real mess, to cover myself really, and he says, oh, he needs no monitor, and I said, are you sure? I still want it, I go by cardiac care asking for a monitor, and I asked the staff nurse if they could monitor, would monitor, or be on the ward, or look after him. No, we can't monitor, she said, no, we can't, and you know, this is the nurse I swear by, but she's having a rough time . . . I said, this guy could arrest. I just needed somebody to bend, to get this guy in . . . and the patient, sure enough, arrived on the ward, arrested and died. Now, I'm not saying you could have prevented it, but we might have seen this rhythm coming along, or whatever but . . . you know, it's horrific.

A similar dichotomy between nursing and medical perspectives can be seen with the discharge of patients from a ward. The consultant wants to empty the beds in order to admit the patients that they have seen in outpatient clinics, and keep their turnover high. Managers want to ensure enough empty beds to provide for emergencies, while also admitting the maximum possible number from the waiting list, a pressure all the more insistent following the introduction of contracts. Ward nursing staff are not usually involved with outpatients, but they have closer contact with ward patients and their relatives than doctors do, so their primary concern is the well-being of the patient on the ward. If they feel a patient is being discharged too early and at risk to their recovery, or in a way that places too great demands on family carers, or before adequate social service support has been organised, they may try to delay discharge. If it is a ward caring for elderly patients needing rehabilitation, the medical aspect of recovery may be less significant than the assessment by physiotherapists, so the ward sister may be representing the views of other professions as well as nursing in trying to delay discharge. Discharge decisions are the responsibility of the consultant, but discharge arrangements have to be undertaken by a named nurse so there is an opportunity for nurses to modify decisions.

> *Nurse manager*: One consultant is keen to keep up a good throughput . . . [Sister] feels he is occasionally a bit too keen to discharge people, whereas she would have given them a little bit longer. So she sometimes just 'forgets' to discharge them.

In short, the doctor's loyalty may be focused on the patients waiting to come into hospital, while the ward nurse gives priority to the patient on the ward. The tensions between these two legitimate concerns can be heightened if nurses feel that the primary aim of a high turnover is to enhance the consultant's or the department's reputation, or if consultants are seen to be admitting so many patients that it becomes impossible to provide good, or even adequate, levels of nursing care. Both nurses and doctors are pressured, but from different directions.

> *Sister*: On numerous occasions they've sent patients home overnight, or admitted them to come in the following morning for theatre because we've run out of beds and in fact we have had 40 patients in 30 beds . . . I think the nursing side is often very stretched to satisfy the needs of doctors because if the number of operations isn't carried out then the surgical committee might remove the registrar.

The tensions about turnover and the need to admit a high number of patients is coloured by a recognition that this has become a highly politicised debate. Information on how many patients are seen by each consultant and how many patients each consultant surgeon treats in any given month are available to the local press and are increasingly commonly reported. While doctors do not overtly change their behaviours as a result of such publicity, it seems likely that the increasingly public arena in which these issues are being discussed has a bearing on the sense of urgency that is attached to the question of admitting greater numbers of patients. Ward nurses, on the other hand, do not figure in such discussions and by tradition and inclination their concern is focused on providing good care for the patients on their ward rather than maximising in every possible way the turnover of new patients. This may change as senior ward sisters are re-born as ward managers and budget holders, seeking to ensure financial survival by completing contract obligations.

Tensions over admissions and discharges relate very closely to funding which is almost entirely outside the control of ward-based staff. Conflicts between medical and nursing staff over admissions occur because each group is representing and seeking to protect a different aspect of health service care. Patients gain from this advocacy, in that no one element of patient care is allowed to dominate. If the devolution of budgets to ward level transforms nurses into advocates of rapid turnover, patients will have lost the adversarial balance that the nursing profession currently brings to this debate.

Communication failure

Hospital wards, in general and teaching hospitals, commonly have 25–30 beds, with average lengths of stay of around three to five days. There are a multiplicity of treatment and care decisions made each day that involve coordinating the work of numerous groups of staff. Doctors and nurses depend on the work of each other to complete their own programme of care or treatment, and effective communication is essential. When this is less than perfect there are problems for each profession.

The largest group of communication failures which were reported to us as causing interprofessional friction were those where the doctor did not tell the nurse something important. If the doctor does not do this then the organisation of the patient for the next day is disrupted as a consequence. For instance, a consultant may come onto the ward, speak to a patient, telling them that they are going home, but does not tell the nursing staff, or they may have ordered some treatment, and put it in the notes, but not informed the nursing staff. A junior doctor who goes off duty and does not pass information to the doctor who is going to be on call can trigger a chain of circumstances that seriously reduces the quality of care and treatment given. A nurse may forget to report to a junior doctor that a patient has been sick or faint, though these could be important symptoms of a changing medical condition.

There are usually three formal mechanisms to provide for exchanges of information: the ward book, the hand-over and the ward round.

Patients' notes and ward day books   The nursing profession emphasises the need meticulously to record patient observations, treatment measures and care plans (UKCC, 1993a). Doctors complain bitterly at times that nurses spend far too much time writing up records at the expense of providing patient care, though a few medical staff report that they use nursing records as a source of useful, accurate and easily accessed information about a patient's condition and home circumstances. There is a continual tension between time to maintain information and notes, and time for patient care.

The ward book is a central record of instructions and decisions on many wards, but inevitably the quality of information given, and the care taken to ensure a comprehensive coverage of information varies from ward to ward. Junior doctors who visit many wards may fume about poor record keeping, but also complain persistently that too much nursing time is spent writing up notes. On an exceptionally busy ward, with an unusual number of patients needing high levels of patient care, time for recording information is at a premium, but it is exactly at such times that information most needs to be exchanged.

The hand-over   This occurs from one shift of nurses to the next, and does not normally involve medical staff. It is a time-consuming but essential exchange of information that involves the shift of nurses coming on duty. Responsibility for each patient is transferred to the nurse coming on duty in order to ensure continuity of care. The hand-over is characteristic of the way that nursing is organised as a team process, while doctors operate much more as autonomous individuals. Doctors who want nursing assistance with some treatment procedure, or who want information about a particular patient, may be exasperated by the time taken by a group of nurses during a hand-over.

There is no equivalent formal process when a house officer hands over to the on-call doctor. Individual doctors vary in the extent to which they pass on information, and this can be so even when a doctor is leaving at the end of a six-month contract. Nursing staff may be so perturbed at the lack of communication that they decide to take some action, but this is well beyond the call of duty. A house officer described what he found on his first day in a new hospital:

> *House officer*: Liz [staff nurse] got the previous houseman to write me a timetable of things to do on the ward, past midnight when he was up, so that when I was coming in I'd get on with it, and . . . I think that's just about the nicest touch I've ever seen. I think the houseman should have done it himself, but, you know, since he didn't, I think that's . . . that's brilliant, I think that's just so considerate.

Many nursing staff express astonishment at the casual way that doctors exchange information, seeing it as an example of lack of professionalism, while medical staff may castigate nurses who spend what is perceived as an undue amount of time on maintaining nursing notes and records.

The ward round   This involves the consultant, the medical team and the sister or senior staff nurse. On some wards therapy staff may join the round, and in teaching hospitals there may be some medical students. This is when the consultant sees the patient, looks at charts, lab reports and X-rays, receives a report on how the patient has responded to treatment, confirms or alters a diagnosis or treatment plan, decides if more investigations are needed, or tells the patient he or she can go home. The ward round is usually a formal and somewhat ritualistic affair. Staff who call each other by their first name will use titles on the ward round. Arguments are reserved for the privacy of the office. A doctor or nurse who has been criticised for some failure will usually suffer in silence.

But the ward round has changed. Staff who have been in post for some time saw the change as remarkable, from the days when patients sat up in bed in regimental rows, counterpanes were turned down the regulation number of inches, the bed wheels all set at right angles to the wall, locker tops gleamed and everything was silenced as the consultant swept in. On wards where there is still a more formal approach nurses see patients having to take second place. The nature of the ward round is determined largely by consultant preferences, so there are marked contrasts between wards. These two staff nurses worked in the same hospital.

> *Staff nurse*: When I first started we didn't have bedpans out on the ward when the consultant was there . . . and you stood by the bed, whereas now life carries on exactly the same . . . if somebody is in the bath when the consultant comes round they will come back to them . . . [patients] won't get hoicked out of the bath because the consultant's due in an hour . . . it's much less formal.

> *Staff nurse*: Consultants . . . come in and stand at the desk and expect you to drop everything and go with them. I think that is probably tradition, it's the way things have always been done, but we are all here for the good of the patient and sometimes I think the patient gets shoved to the back.

An informal ward round means that patients' needs do not have to be ignored, and precious nursing time is not lost, but it does increase the chances of some exchange of information being missed. Many instructions are given verbally. If a doctor sees a patient individually, and not as part of the ward round, the patient may be the only person on the ward aware of the doctor's decision, and blissfully unaware of the need to ensure that the nursing staff share that information.

Visits from consultant medical staff that are not part of a formal ward round are normal practice if there are several consultants with patients on one ward. This is most likely in a teaching hospital, both because of the number of consultants and because emergency admissions are likely to be distributed over many wards.

Number of consultants   The number of consultants working in each ward varies considerably, from the traditional one consultant to one ward pattern to the situation found in some teaching hospitals where, we were told, it was not uncommon to have the patients of a dozen consultants on one ward; having 20 consultants' patients at one time was not unknown. At one of the hospitals we visited management and medical staff were considering breaking the link between consultants and beds for each specialty, so that a surgical patient could be assigned a bed on any surgical ward, and each surgeon would have patients on each ward, with similar systems for other specialties.

Each consultant has junior doctors, so ward sisters and staff nurses have to receive and relate information to a considerable number of doctors. With a large number of consultants each one cannot take up the time of a senior nurse with a formal ward round. Nor does the consultant easily find time to programme each visit to each ward on a set timetable. Ward rounds are timetabled for the consultant's 'base' ward, and other patients are seen when it is convenient for senior medical staff. The ward sister keeps an eye open for consultants 'popping in', to try to catch them before they go, to see what has been decided. On some wards it is the junior doctor, not the consultant who needs to be watched:

> *Sister*: Sometimes when they are going to the car park, or on the way to the bank or to lunch, they'll say maybe 'oh, we'll whiz on before we go to lunch', and the patient might be near the door, round the front – because that's where the higher dependency patients are – and they just whiz off again. And then you have to go round and say to the patient 'well, what did the doctor say to you?' . . . [or] we get told about it from the patient, or the X-ray department or whoever will ring up and say 'by the way, did you know that . . .' and you then can't really be bothered to go out of your way a bit to make sure things are done, because there are certain doctors . . . you get to know who is like that. The patient doesn't get treated quite so well because of that kind of poor contact.

The difficulty of finding a nurse who is not busy with a patient is such that this also adds to the chance of the doctor disappearing without exchanging information. Ward clerical staff provide an information base, but such staff may be non-existent, or only work for limited hours. However, the large number of consultants involved on any particular ward is often linked to having 'outlier' or 'boarded out' patients.

Outliers Patients variously known as 'lodgers', 'boarders' or 'outliers' are those who are being nursed on wards which are organised for a different specialty. They are an 'outlier' for the specialty firm which admitted them. This situation exists because of a need to admit emergency patients to whichever ward has a bed vacancy, which may be on a ward not at all connected to the consultant's specialty. The practice of having outliers is one response to the pressure that emerged in the 1970s to utilise hospital beds more efficiently, by increasing bed occupancy rates and improving turnover while reducing the overall number of hospital beds.

Some wards are more likely than others to have outlier patients because they have a higher proportion of minor surgical cases. On wards where many patients are sent home by the weekend, and new patients don't arrive for operations until Monday, there are empty beds at the weekend which can be used for emergency admissions if other surgical or medical wards are full. Some consultants have a firm policy of getting patients back to their base ward if at all possible, while others prefer not to move the patients so that they can build up a relationship with nursing staff.

One effect of having 'outliers' is that junior doctors, house officers and SHOs, have to visit a considerable number of wards in order to see their consultant's patients. Treatment and management plans have to be arranged with nurses who do not necessarily have appropriate specialist skills, who do not know the junior doctor, and who want the patient moved in order to be able to admit 'their' patients from the waiting list for surgical operations. For a junior doctor walking in to yet another unfamiliar ward, it is tempting to nip on to the ward, see the patient, and avoid the hassle of having to deal with a set of unknown and potentially hostile nurses, who may not go out of their way to be welcoming. By contrast, a ward where the nursing staff are known, and their skills and competence recognised, will become a base for house officers, and inevitably a place where there is better exchange of patient information, and better teamworking.

> *Sister*: We usually tend to have quite a close working relationship with the housemen based on the ward, I suppose because they're here most of the time, they tend to use the facilities, they have coffee and things, whereas the ones from outside the ward don't feel like it's their base.

All hospitals find it necessary to place patients on inappropriate wards, especially during winter months when the number of patients admitted as medical emergencies may exceed the number of medical ward beds, so that medical patients have to be nursed on surgical wards. (Patients waiting for surgery have their operations deferred.) Newer hospitals may be designed in ways that allow easy access between medical and surgical wards, so there is an in-built flexibility in the way that beds can be managed. Smaller hospitals also have less of a problem because no ward is very remote, and there is a better chance of knowing someone on each ward. In a large teaching hospital patients may be quite distant and all the nursing staff unknown. The practice of having to work in many wards is one of the reasons why house officers and SHOs expressed a strong preference for life in a district general hospital (DGH). A junior doctor contrasted his first house officer post in a DGH with his second posting in a teaching hospital:

SHO: In [the DGH] I was based on one ward, there was one sister, and there were a couple of staff nurses who had been there a long time and were very experienced . . . you soon get to know each other very well, and you work as a team. In [the teaching hospital], my second house job, obviously when I was at a similar level, I was working on, maybe, at various times, anything up to eight wards . . . and so, you are being bleeped constantly, everybody's frustrated, 'cause you're spending time on this ward and that ward and the other ward, and you don't get to know the staff . . .

The dilemma that increasing bed occupancy results in fragmentation of the ward team has long been recognised in the health management literature (Dowling and Barrett, 1991; Marshall and Spencer, 1974; Yates, 1982). Increasing the numbers of outliers is a response to pressure, but creates pressure elsewhere. Bed occupancy is a highly visible performance indicator for management, while quality of patient care and the morale of staff is less a matter of concern. More importantly, there is little evidence of attention being given to determining whether the quality of care or the outcome of treatment is significantly reduced when patients are nursed on inappropriate wards.

Primary nursing and ward rounds   The introduction of primary nursing is another reason why the ward round in its traditional form is becoming obsolete on some wards. Primary nursing is a system of allocating a small number of patients to the care of a named nurse. Over a succession of shifts the patient receives nursing care from their named nurses. The ward sister's role is to support and advise the primary nurse, but not to take over responsibility for managing the patient. It is a reform in patient care that has been introduced by the nursing profession, and supported through the Patient's Charter. Where primary nursing has been introduced it has generally been warmly welcomed by patients. It has also shown itself to be a reform that is influential in changing the working patterns and relationships of professional staff. Primary nursing is in keeping with a central notion of 'new wave' management, of bringing responsibility for service delivery close to the customer. Interestingly, it is a management reform that is professionally led, and derives from a professional service ethos.

For doctors the initial impact of primary nursing is disturbing. No longer is the ward sister able to provide a single point of reference. To find out how twelve patients are progressing it may be necessary to approach three different nurses, none of them as senior as the ward sister. At the time of our interviews there were only a handful of wards using a primary nursing system, but doctors who had adjusted to the new system were realising that there were advantages for them, in that primary nurses are closer to their patients, and therefore better informed about the patients' condition than it is possible for a ward sister to be. The disadvantage for consultants is that they do not know the primary nurse, who may be a grade of nurse with little previous experience of working directly with a consultant or senior registrar. Primary nursing requires an acceptance that the familiar information flow along the hierarchy of ward sister to consultant has to be modified.

In spite of the advantage of improved information, some consultants are not willing to make adjustments to the traditional ward round. A nursing officer described the reaction of two consultants to the introduction of teamworking, a modified form of primary care.

> *Nursing officer*: The consultant up here has accepted team nursing . . . he is quite happy to do the ward round with the team leader, even if she is an enrolled nurse . . . he's found he gets more knowledge about the patients because the team leaders are more involved than the ward sister was. On the ward downstairs the consultant really wants to do his ward round with the sister and if she is not there we have a problem . . . he really likes it to be quiet and everybody ready for him and the nursing staff to actually help him doing his ward round . . . that is very difficult because really we are moving in a different direction.

Medical staff need to know whether treatment is working or, if a patient is getting worse, what signs and symptoms of deterioration have been noted. Nurses who have more contact with patients are likely to have some of that information. Patient care reduces in quality if either a nurse is not available to discuss the patient with the doctor, or a doctor is not willing to absorb information proffered by a nurse.

Formal communication mechanisms are only part of the communication process. Throughout the day and frequently at night doctors call on the ward for one task and are given a string of other messages. How they deal with these is a significant factor. Consultants are usually on the ward less frequently than junior staff, and information exchange is more formal. Consultants have been particularly strong in expressing both the importance of informal information and the difficulty of maintaining the links that make such exchanges possible. The practice of having coffee after the ward round has often been discarded, and effective information exchange is harder to bring about when there is minimal opportunity for informal contact. It is perhaps more surprising that so much information is processed effectively than it is that there are significant failures at times.

In Chapter 2 we provided a simplified chart of ward accountability (Figure 2.2, p. 35). The process of information exchange between ward nursing and medical staff is far more complex than that chart might suggest. Primary nursing significantly alters the way that patient information is exchanged. The adjustments that medical staff have to make to accommodate primary nursing are compensated for by the benefits that they receive. The level of information is likely to be better, and there is a flexibility that does not exist with formal ward rounds. The traditional ward round system does not work well when there are a large number of consultants with patients on each ward. Primary nurses who are closely identified with a small number of patients can potentially provide an effective communication base for exchanging essential information, that is better suited to the wards with numerous medical teams (see Figure 4.1).

Bleeps

A specific aspect of communication in hospitals is the use of the pager or bleep. Bleeps were introduced about 20 years ago to overcome the communication problems caused by having medical and nursing staff working in different locations. It was assumed that this would create more efficient working by enabling doctors to be rapidly called to where they were most needed. Before bleeps were introduced, nurses rang around the wards and residences. Now doctors can be contacted with a level of surety that was not possible before. There are few nurses who carry bleeps; until recently, this was only likely to happen in particular specialisms so that nurses typically do not experience the intrusive nature of bleeps.

What the bleep has done is to transfer a significant part of the frustration of working in different locations from the nurse to the doctor. Before the introduction of bleeps nurses spent much valuable time trying to locate the doctor. Now nurses can get a message to the doctor relatively easily, and the doctor has to find a phone to ring back in response to a bleep. The frustration for the doctor has increased massively. For the nurse the irritation is in waiting for the doctor to respond.

Many junior doctors are adamant that, far from increasing efficiency, the bleep reduces efficiency because a large number of unnecessary calls prevent them from organising their work effectively, and add unacceptable levels of stress by making it impossible to eat a meal, talk to a colleague, or even go to the bathroom without interruption. In an article entitled 'Slaves to the hospital bleep' one junior doctor expresses her intense dislike of the bleep in terms that match exactly with the information we derived from our interviews with junior doctors.

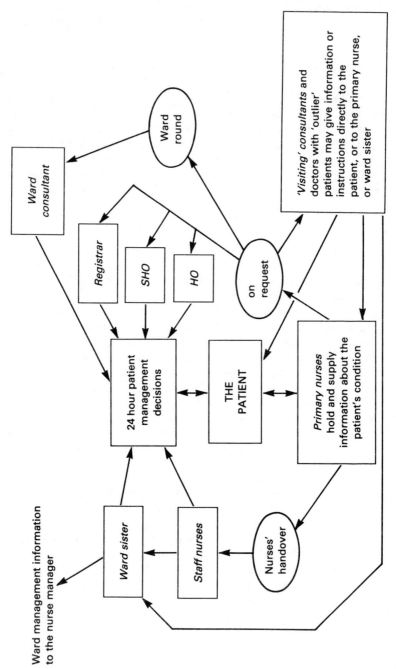

Figure 4.1 *Primary nursing and information exchange (the arrows denote information flow)*

The most despised object is the bleep. It constantly interrupts a day's work. Introduced to improve efficiency, it now does the opposite . . . the bleep is seen as a quick fix, and no regard is paid to the disruption it causes. The immediacy and ease of the bleep system have led to its excessive use. (*Guardian*, 25 September 1991)

> *House officer*: Instead of being left in peace and being able to organise our work as we want to we are at the mercy of our pagers. Instead of being used as they were initially conceived for as a way of contacting doctors in an emergency, they are used for every single pathetic problem that is at hand. That is a major bone of contention.

Apart from some consultants, all doctors carry bleeps so that they can be summoned when needed. When staff are bleeped they are supposed to find the nearest phone and call in. Most frequently it is junior doctors who are called out by staff nurses. Doctors up to consultant level may be on call for many more hours than they are working, but for a consultant or senior registrar, being called out happens significantly less frequently than for junior doctors. Also they will be called by the junior doctor, while it is nurses who call the house officers or SHOs.

Both nurses and doctors reported conflict over the issues relating to the use of the bleep, but the nature of their comments were markedly different (Mackay, 1993). Many junior doctors complain bitterly that nurses bleep them unnecessarily about stupid things, or that more than one nurse bleeps them about the same thing. That there are occasions of genuine inappropriate bleeping is evidenced by the fact that nurses also report their embarrassment at the way that nursing colleagues bleep doctors.

> *Sister*: I don't think that I will ever forget it, they bleeped the doctor at 3 o'clock in the morning to say that this lady's blood sugar result had come back, and it was four days prior to this that this blood sugar result had come back . . . he was so angry, and . . . I can understand that.

A related issue is where the ward is organised for primary nursing, so there are different nurses responsible for different patients, and each one bleeps the house officer about their particular patient – on the same ward. Nurses insist that this never happens, junior doctors are adamant that it does. While there is some sympathy for a young doctor at everyone's beck and call, there is also a feeling among nurses that some doctors have only themselves to blame because they do not anticipate problems, or prepare prescriptions or instructions in advance.

Nurses commonly complained that doctors were slow to arrive when bleeped, but only rarely that they did not arrive at all.

Sometimes doctors may be delayed because they are too busy, too lazy or too exhausted from lack of sleep to care. From the nurse's viewpoint there is the fury when a doctor does not appear after being bleeped and does not even ring in. A refusal to come at all when bleeped is regarded as being quite different from taking a long time to come because the doctor has other priorities, and is regarded very seriously by both the nursing and medical hierarchy. It is seen as neglect of duty, rather than generating tension over priorities. The failure to come at all when bleeped made nurses very angry. Occasionally sisters have reported ringing up the consultant when a house officer or SHO has failed to come. The consultant who then rings the junior doctor regards the failure to arrive as a serious situation . . . If the junior doctor is not working properly then the nurses make sure the consultant knows, often via the registrar. On night duty the nurse manager will often take responsibility for putting pressure on a junior doctor who is refusing to turn out.

> *Nurse manager*: My last set of nights . . . the nurse in charge had difficulty in getting [the house officer] to come and see a patient who had a tachycardia (fast pulse) of 156 . . . So I phoned him and said, basically, if you are not happy at coming I will phone your registrar, whereupon he came.

Doctors frequently complain that they are bleeped merely so that the nurse can write 'doctor informed' in the notes and not for a substantive medical reason, or that when they do arrive on the ward in response to a bleep, the nurse immediately uses the doctor's arrival as an opportunity to see to another patient rather than engaging in a dialogue with the doctor. This is behaviour that the doctor sees as unprofessional, or further evidence of the 'doctor informed' syndrome, whereas to nurses with many patients to see to it is a reasonable response since the doctor is capable of seeing to the ill patient him/herself. On a busy ward, communication may be seen as less of a priority than meeting patient care needs, but leaving a doctor to deal with a patient can imply that the knowledge that the nurse holds about a patient's condition is not highly valued by the nurse themselves.

On the other side, nurses frequently complain that doctors will not listen to what they do say, so creating an incentive to say little above what is absolutely necessary. They bleep the doctor and then write 'doctor informed' in the notes because they must as part of their strict procedures and in order to cover themselves. This is a product of nurses' relationship to their own hierarchy and, whether or not they like this, they often have little choice about the limits of their conduct. Bleeping and writing 'doctor informed' is part of a rule conscious practice, but if the particular doctor and nurse have a good working relationship then they may be able to cooperate more fully than this, so making more effective and economical use of the doctor's time.

Whatever system is set up, the individual doctor and nurse must be able to rely on each other's competence for the system to work well. A comment from several junior doctors was that they need to know the capabilities of individual nurses since they varied so much in competence and style of practice. It was a commonly held opinion that rule breaking was necessary for satisfactory working relationships, provided it was based on trust in the competence of colleagues. This can only develop if staff have worked together sufficiently often to have made an informal assessment of the quality of the other's work. Falling back on the minimalism of the rules is both safer, and inevitable if staff do not know each other's capabilities. Effective cooperation requires a stable team, but some of the methods needed to maximise hospital 'efficiency' reduce the likelihood that ward staff will be working with familiar colleagues. Short contracts for junior doctors have a similar impact. The question of the bleep is compounded when it comes when the doctor is exhausted and is snatching a few hours of sleep. The long hours worked by most junior doctors is a crucial issue here; they may be on call from 8 a.m. Friday to 5 p.m. the following Monday.

The bleep is a surprisingly complex issue. It is partly a dispute over whether tasks are simple enough for nurses to do, with the implication that they should do them and not call on the more valuable time of the doctor; that is, it is a version of the hierarchical relationship between the professions. It is partly a problem of the fuzziness of the boundary between diagnosis and care in that any change in the course of treatment is considered to be solely the province of the doctor, but the differential exposure of doctors and nurses to professional and legal censure is also a factor. Nurses call out doctors even if they think they know the appropriate course of action because if they make a mistake they are liable to overt professional disciplinary procedures. If they step over the boundary between diagnosis and care they risk severe penalties. But essentially the bleep is an indicator of the fragmentation of the ward team by the time–space geography of hospital organisation, a fragmentation that is increased by demands for maximal use of the hospital's resources, and made more acute by a lack of concern for the impact on more junior medical and nursing staff.

Effective teams

Summary of influential factors
There is no one factor that can ensure that effective nurse–doctor teams exist. The data we collected indicated a variety of factors that increased or diminished the likelihood that effective teams would emerge. These are summarised in Table 4.4. The mixture of several factors seems more important than the presence of any one element. So, for example, staff with a high commitment to good patient care, who have been in post for some time, and who have a high regard for each other's competence, may be able successfully to manage the tensions of working in a multi-consultant ward with a strong research and teaching tradition, and which is frequently used for outlier patients from other specialties.

A stable nursing staff is usually a positive factor in interprofessional relations. But in some circumstances the existence within a hospital of a high percentage of senior ward nursing staff in post for many years can have a different impact. Medical staff attitudes, funding pressures and nursing philosophies can combine to produce a pervasive sense of each profession digging in its heels to maintain the boundaries of its professional territory. For example, in a situation where there is a long-standing disagreement over appropriate nurse staffing levels, combined with a medical commitment to research and teaching, and a medical determination to control the nursing agenda, then the response of nursing staff is one of active resistance rather than cooperation. In this situation, the existence of a core of nursing colleagues with some years of work at the same hospital provides mutual support that reinforces nurse solidarity and resistance to medical domination.

Hospital and specialty differences
The extent of hospital variation was striking, especially between the extremes of Greenfield and College hospitals. The variation between these two hospitals was noticeable throughout and raises important questions as to why patterns of interprofessional relations should vary so much. The research design had been linked to an expectation of specialty, professional and gender differences. A hospital effect had not been anticipated. Interestingly, Carr-Hill et al. (1992) also found some evidence of a hospital effect, but no consistent difference between medical and surgical wards. The information available from interviews does not allow for a definitive analysis, but there is sufficient evidence to suggest probable explanations.

Table 4.4 lists a variety of factors that have a positive or negative

Table 4.4 *Factors influencing effective ward teams*

	Positive factors	Negative factors
Admission policies, staffing levels	Ward nurse staffing levels compatible with medical staff admission and discharge policy	Inadequate coordination between nurse staffing levels and admission discharge policy
Number of consultants	A small number of consultants based on the ward. Few 'visiting' consultants	A multi-consultant ward; or one frequently used for 'outlier' patients
Staffing stability	Ward sister and staff nurses in post for several years. Minimal use of locum medical staff. Bank and agency nurses employed who are well known to permanent staff	High turnover of nursing staff. Frequent employment of medical locums. Much use of agency nurses unfamiliar with the ward
Commitment to quality	A strong commitment to high-quality patient care by both professions	Low commitment to high-quality treatment or care, or medical priority is given to teaching and research
Junior staff roles	The relative status of house officers and nursing staff is clearly defined	House officers/SHOs do not respect nursing expertise. Nurses close off any dialogue with junior medical staff
Primary nursing	A well-established primary nursing system	Introducing a primary nursing system
Respected colleagues	Mutual recognition of professional competence	Mistrust of the skill of senior medical or nursing colleagues
Staff support systems	Responsiveness to reports of staff inadequacies	Will not confront staff failures reported by another profession
Consultant involvement	Consultant involvement in ward management issues, but with recognition of areas of nursing autonomy	'Absentee' or uninterested consultant, or nursing staff who exclude the consultant from ward management policy
Nursing leadership	Nursing control of nursing budgets	Unassertive nursing staff. Medical control of nursing
Task negotiation	Flexible task boundaries. Negotiated agreement of responsibilities	Medical dumping of unwanted tasks on nurses. Nurses insist on rigid task boundaries

effect on good teamworking. Some of these patterns are relevant to Greenfield and College. Greenfield is a district general hospital, College is a teaching hospital. Greenfield had several wards with a single consultant, and none with the array of numerous consultants found in some teaching hospital wards. The smaller size of the hospital, and the building design, made the management of outlier patients relatively straightforward. Greenfield was also free of the tensions generated by medical research and teaching commitments. Both hospitals had a low turnover of nursing staff.

So far we have discussed aspects that are within what could be considered a professional management agenda. However, some of the factors which are most likely to be relevant in producing a different hospital culture and organisation lie outside the control of hospital staff. This is especially the case with funding levels. In the 1980s the position of the hospital in relation to regional reallocations of funding was an important factor. During this decade funding to district health authorities was weighted to compensate for historical imbalances between geographical areas. The formula used to allocate funding targets was known as RAWP (Resource Allocation Working Party). The hospitals involved in our study had had significantly varying positions in relation to RAWP reallocation of funding.

Greenfield had the most advantageous RAWP position and Greenfield staff recognised that they were in a better position than many other hospitals. During interviews staff noted that they had 'escaped the worst of the cuts', though few proffered any explanation of this statement.

College had had several years of receiving a less favourable RAWP budget. Typically, staff do not cut the number of services when their funding position is less advantageous. For some years they strive to maintain the same range of services, with each specialty getting a relatively less generous budget. The tensions this process generates emerges in several of the accounts of conflicts over admissions, theatre budgets and ward nurse staffing. Not all of these are from College; funding generated tensions in all hospitals, but to a markedly lesser extent at Greenfield than at College.

Funding pressures are most visible in relation to nurse staffing, but they have a significant impact on the way the hospital is organised as a whole to maximise 'output'. To gain extra funds from discretionary allocations, hospital managers have to show that they are achieving targets for reducing waiting lists, managing a high throughput of patients, and maintaining appropriately high bed occupancy rates. To achieve these aims it has often been necessary to rationalise the use of hospital facilities, a process that usually necessitates closing some wards, or smaller hospitals, and concentrating services on fewer sites. A rationalisation process of this kind can fragment existing teams, and is usually dispiriting in its effect on staff. Central and County hospitals were in the midst of rationalisation programmes at the time of our interviews. City had completed the first stage of a reorganisation of elderly care wards before interviews began.

Rationalising bed usage means using existing facilities more intensively. Quite apart from the impact on those wards most directly affected by changes in service provision, there is operational pressure on all wards because of the reduced number of beds available to deal with emergencies. There is continual need to achieve a higher turnover, and maintain a downward pressure on costs, without diminishing the quality of care and treatment. The fault-lines that run between the professions become more evident under this kind of pressure.

At Greenfield, rationalisation of local hospital services had meant the closure of older buildings some years earlier, and the concentration of services on a single site within a newly built hospital. Many of the staff had worked together for several years in the older hospitals and had also been at Greenfield long enough to form new professional loyalties.

Our tentative explanation for the contrast between Greenfield and College has therefore several elements. Greenfield interviews took place at a time when the probability of good teamwork was high. Funding pressures existed, but were manageable without being destructive. Rationalisation had been achieved a few years previously by being able to concentrate services in a new hospital, rather than having to use existing buildings more intensively. There had been time to settle down after the move. The size of the hospital, the way that wards were organised, the presence of wards with a single consultant, and the low turnover of hospital nursing staff and consultants were all features conducive to good teamwork. Tensions were most evident in connection with the boundaries of professional responsibilities rather than over admissions or theatre budgets.

At College, professional boundary tensions were evident alongside the pressures generated by tight service budgets continuing for some years. As described earlier, funding pressures influence professional cooperation. There were, though, other cultural factors that were evident, but impossible to explain adequately. Questions about socialising off duty showed that in all four of the five hospitals, fewer doctors and nurses met socially than the common image of the professions would suggest. At College the distance between the two groups was particularly marked. A small example was given by an SHO, who reported that she was the only one of 40 doctors who accepted an invitation to the A&E department's nursing staff Christmas 'night out'. The media image of 'casualty' is very different from this.

Effective teams: an example of good practice
The evidence that funding pressure is a significant element affecting professional teamwork is substantial, but other factors are also relevant. To focus on these we have selected a department which reported good teamwork to an extent that was untypical of the hospital as a whole. That is, its effective teamworking could not be explained by levels of funding. The most noticeable example is the surgical department at Central hospital (see Table A1, Appendix A, p. 183).

The response from Central hospital surgical department stands out for three reasons: it is significantly more positive than would have been predicted by looking at the responses from surgical departments in the other four hospitals; it is more positive than other departments at Central hospital; and it is accompanied by reports of not infrequent conflict. Almost all the staff in this department considered that they worked well as a team, in spite of having overt and sometimes intense disagreements. This raises the question of what respondents meant when reporting good medical–nursing teamwork.

Careful examination of interview transcripts showed that several features associated with good medical/nursing relationships were present. There were consistent references to the competence of the consultants and the ward sisters. Nursing staff had been in post for some time. There were few consultants involved on particular wards, and the small size of the department, and the nature of inter-consultant relationships, made it possible to maximise bed usage without producing conflict. One noticeable and unusual factor was the frequency with which nursing staff referred to the approach-ability of the consultants, and the emphasis in the consultant interview on welcoming overt questioning of medical issues by nurses. This was about to be formalised by involving nurses in medical case discussions. It was not at all linked to any weakening of medical control of treatment; there was a continuing conflict over wound management that looked likely to be settled by referring all treatment decisions to the consultant. Ultimate medical control did not, though, mean that the views of nursing staff were ignored.

There was also evidence of intraprofessional support. The nursing profession is often poor in giving support to colleagues and the existence of a supportive intraprofessional network in this instance may have worked in a positive way to encourage a rather more informal interprofessional style. There were sufficient numbers of nurses with extended role qualifications to ensure that the management of IV fluids was not a contentious issue with junior medical and nursing staff. On the occasions when house officers caused conflict with nursing staff by their attitude, the consultant typically identified with the nursing staff viewpoint. Only the position of the locum registrar was more problematic, and senior medical staff had been called on by nurses to override the treatment decisions of locum registrars, creating an exception to the generally good working relations in this unit.

In the opinion of the consultant, good teamworking was noticeable wherever there was a high level of emergency surgery, in contrast to departments that concentrated on 'cold' surgery (i.e. admission of patients from a waiting list). Central hospital surgery had a large element of emergency work. The priority of medical and nursing staff was identical: the rapid and effective treatment of patients.

The overall picture is of a department that is committed to good quality care, where both medical and nursing staff are assertive, confident, and respective of each other's contribution, where nursing staff are able to accommodate different consultant styles without weakening their own professional agenda, and where senior medical and nursing staff have been in post long enough to form effective teams. The existence of conflict over professional boundary issues did not override the strengths of the permanent staff team, but did require continuing interprofessional management.

Conclusion

Nearly half the points of conflict between doctors and nurses can be traced back to the fragmentation of the time–space geography of the hospital under pressure. This disintegration of the ward as an organic unit has caused many problems. In particular, it makes the exchange of information between doctors and nurses much more difficult: it becomes more liable to error, which causes conflict. The bleep is a focus of some of these frustrations over the effort to communicate. The fragmentation makes what would otherwise be minor issues over nurses not maintaining IVs, or administering minor painkillers, into major frustrations on occasion. The pressure on resources is partly the reason here, combined with an increase in medical specialism. There is also the question of whether the need for an information policy giving priority to the fast accurate exchange of information between doctors and nurses takes second place to the managerial drive to increase turnover rates.

In order to understand the reasons behind good teamworking and those situations where it breaks down, we need to analyse the pressure on resources, how these are managed and the management of interprofessional relations. The wider factors influencing these outcomes include: the tension along the boundary between the professions (see Chapter 3); the tension between different modes of management (see Chapter 5); and the tension between Fordism and post-Fordism (see Chapter 6).

We began this chapter by discussing briefly how ward level staff are positioned within Taylorist and 'new wave' schools of management theory. There are particular frustrations in discussing these issues after interviewing hospital nurses and doctors in 1990–91. The strong impression from the data we collected was that the NHS was organised along the lines of a Taylorist management structure. Ward-based teams were not the focus of concern, and were sometimes fragmented in the search for cost-effective and 'efficient' ways of managing hospitals.

However, at the time that interviews were being conducted, NHS hospitals were facing the challenge of preparing to implement the 1991 reforms. These reforms contain specific proposals to devolve power to medical specialties, and then to wards. The direction of change was therefore, theoretically at least, moving towards a much greater concern to strengthen ward-based teams at precisely the time when we were hearing of the fragmentation of ward teams. Clinical directorates, which are discussed in the next chapter, were being planned, and the devolution of budgets to a ward level was under discussion.

There is, though, no indication that maximising turnover of patients and maintaining pressure on costs will be any less of a priority. The stress on working relationships caused by budget pressure seems likely to continue. If devolution of decision making is genuinely a matter of concern, then the question of how to strengthen and maintain interprofessional teams will have to be afforded much greater priority. Strengthening the management structure in the NHS was necessary to underpin the introduction of general management, and then to face the challenge of introducing a market mechanism. Strengthening patient-based staff teams is of equal or more importance when the focus is on the benefits of devolving responsibility downwards.

5

Managing Professionals

The fragmentation of the care and treatment of a patient into the hands of many different health workers creates difficulties both for interprofessional relations and for patients. This fragmentation is the negative side of the process of specialisation that most experts on the management of employment otherwise advocate. However, management approaches differ as to the appropriate degree of specialisation and the ways in which this can be balanced by processes of reintegration. The previous chapter showed the tensions produced by these processes of fragmentation in the context of increasing pressure to treat and care for more patients.

While perceived scarcity of resources is common to most health care systems, there are competing approaches as to how to achieve their best optimum use (Davis et al., 1990; Saltman and von Otter, 1992). In some approaches centralisation and tightly specified rules are seen as the route to coordination and productivity. In others, decentralisation and autonomy are seen as the way to increase productivity. On the one hand, fragmentation, while regrettable, may be seen none the less as a worthwhile price to pay for the efficiencies generated by the fuller use of resources and greater specialisation. On the other hand, the greater cohesion of the work team is seen as more productive because it encourages greater worker commitment and enables the development of more rounded knowledge of the process at the centre of concern.

Recent management literature has divided into two main approaches to these dilemmas: Taylorism, sometimes known as scientific management; and 'new wave' management, sometimes known as human resource management. Taylorism has focused on strong central control and the sub-division of tasks in order to increase efficiency, while new wave management, such as that described and advocated by Peters and Waterman (1982), has stressed the importance of engaging worker commitment in order to get the most productive work done. New wave management theory itself contains a tension between a more holistic approach to work so as to make it more meaningful and to engage commitment, and decentralisation which, while producing autonomy, may fragment functions and work relations.

Decentralisation may be only down to the board level of a subsidiary unit, and not to the workers who produce the goods or services. It is thus possible to have a form of Taylorism that gives a cadre of management staff greater autonomy in line with new wave principles, but demands that they utilise Taylorist principles in managing staff. We find it useful to refer to this pattern as devolved Taylorism. For professional staff this is 'macho management'. For the proponents of an energised personnel function, it is having the courage to 'take on the professions', and rationalise professional staffing profiles in order to achieve substantial cost reductions with which to fund improved service provision. Peters and Waterman's stress on engaging worker commitment is less in evidence than a process of rationalising the workforce.

Taylorism and new wave management are thus competing theories as to the best way to manage human resources. They may coexist, for instance, being used by the same employer for different sections of the workforce. Indeed, Atkinson (1986) has developed a model in which the workforce is divided into a core and a periphery, the core being managed by engaging workers' commitment, and the periphery by sub-division of tasks and casualisation.

These approaches are to be found in parallel in management theory and in the sociology of employment, and, further, they have significant resonance in wider theories of societal organisation. In the sociology of employment there are analyses of Taylorism by writers, such as Braverman (1974), who see it as the managerial logic of contemporary capitalism. This compares with accounts by Elger (1979) and by Freidman (1977) who have argued that responsible autonomy was an equally successful way of managing the workforce.

Social theorists have placed these analyses of the changing organisation of employment within broader theories of changes in society as a whole (see Aglietta, 1987; Drucker, 1993; Piore and Sabel, 1984). These broader issues of social change will be addressed in Chapter 6.

This chapter will argue for the utility of assessing management theory alongside the sociology of employment to analyse the professions. Then it will consider the divergent strands of management theory. It will interpret some of the points of tension between our two professions described in earlier chapters in the light of the contradictions between forms of management practice. Next we will consider the relationship of traditional notions of professionalism to the different management theories, arguing that the mode of governance of traditional professions has some striking similarities with the prescriptions of new wave management, although there are some divergences.

The management of professions

The coordination of the work of professionals is typically considered separately from that of non-professional workers. This special treatment is misplaced and prevents a full understanding of the organisation of this work. For instance, it mistakenly sets up professional workers apart from and indeed against managerial workers.

What is management? This is not obvious in the organisation of health work. Popularly, it might be thought that management is that work which is done by people called managers and is to do with the organisation and regulation of the work of other workers. In fact, administrators sit uneasily within the category of management, since the presumption is that administrators implement policy on behalf of another group or person, rather than create policy themselves. The conventional picture of the internal organisation of professions is that this is somehow not management. Management is other than professional work. The two categories are seen as mutually exclusive and opposed. Management is about money and resources; bureaucracy and rules; committees and paperwork. Professional work is about treatment and caring; codes of conduct and training; mutual respect for competence and negotiation of any difficulties (see Flynn, 1990; Stacey, 1988).

However, it is wrong to think that management is only carried out by those people with the title of manager. Rather, many doctors and nurses are also managers. They are managers in three ways: first, senior members of each profession organise, monitor and regulate the work of people more junior than themselves in each profession, secondly, they organise patients, thirdly, some of them organise, monitor and regulate the work of people in other occupations. Most notably here, consultants and sometimes other doctors set parameters of treatment and care which organise the work of nurses. Further, we have already seen that doctors and nurses mutually monitor and attempt to regulate certain aspects of each other's work.

The organisation of the professions needs to be considered as a mode of management in its own right. Both medicine and nursing have internal hierarchies in which senior professionals organise, monitor and regulate the work of junior members. They have national professional associations which set down rules of conduct to which their members must conform if they are to retain the right to practise their profession. These are endorsed by the state. In medicine this is the General Medical Council (GMC) and in nursing the United Kingdom Central Council for Nursing, Midwifery and Health Visiting (UKCC). The GMC and UKCC are recognised by the state as the appropriate bodies to license medical and nursing practitioners respectively. In addition, there are further professional associations which act as significant pressure groups, the British Medical Association (BMA), the Royal Colleges associated with each major medical specialty, the Royal College of Nursing, as well as the trade unions representing wider ranges of health workers, notably the former Confederation of Health Service Employees (COHSE) and National Union of Public Employees (NUPE), recently amalgamated into UNISON. The GMC and UKCC effectively regulate the labour market in medical and nursing practitioners since, without their approval, no one can practise as a doctor or nurse.

All labour markets need to be regulated to enforce standards, accountability and efficiency. All systems of regulation need to say something about standards of technical competence and ethics; whether practitioners are obliged to give an account of their actions and if so to whom; and the extent to which the efficiency of practitioners is relevant for regulation. There are four tasks for regulation to control: market entry and exit (from highly permissive to highly restrictive); competitive practices (preventing fraud, enforcing contracts, etc.); market organisation (what kinds of institutions are to be allowed to provide the services, what structure of ownership is permitted); and remuneration (scales of charges, what can and cannot be charged to whom) (Majone, 1990; Moran and Wood, 1993).

> Professionalism is a form of occupational control, a way of regulating the market in a job through controls over entry, over competitive practices, over market structures and over payment. This regulation is done with the agreement of the state, but the form of that agreement – the amount of state supervision, the exact content of the rules – varies over time and in different countries . . . Regulation is political: the institutions that develop, and the rules that those institutions enforce, are produced by the exercise of power. (Moran and Wood, 1993: 27)

Management theories

There are different models of management, as noted above: first, the conventional Taylorist model; secondly, new wave management, popularised by Peters and Waterman (1982); thirdly, the core–periphery model of Atkinson (1986) and the shamrock model of Handy (1990) which both attempt to combine the first two.

Under Taylorism, or scientific management, the management goal is to extract more output from workers by a series of tight control mechanisms. Work is highly monitored and supervised. Wages are considered to be the major incentive for hard work, combined with tight supervision. Complex tasks are broken down into simpler ones so that less skilled and lower paid workers can be employed. There is a separation of the conception and design of the work from its execution, so that management can better direct and control the workers. There is a tight and direct management hierarchy, with power firmly located at the top.

New wave, or human resource management, has a different set of assumptions around which its theory and practice are based. It presumes that workers can become committed to their work for reasons not directly related to wages and that this is the key to more effective organisational coordination. The agenda of new wave management is often seen to revolve around the need to understand the significance of management culture and the need for this story to be one of creativity and constant change if the company is to be successful. Rather than having narrowly and tightly defined roles, jobs are more loosely and flexibly defined.

The highly influential text by Peters and Waterman (1982) *In Search of Excellence* is usually seen to have set the new wave management agenda (Wood, 1989). Peters and Waterman argue that the best US companies share the following eight characteristics:

1 A bias for action, rather than the over-complexities of structure and quantitative techniques learnt in business school; an eagerness to experiment.
2 Close involvement with customers so they know what they want, and to be sensitive to what they will buy.
3 Autonomy and entrepreneurship within the company, the support of product champions and mavericks, to enable innovation to continue.
4 Productivity through people, recognising that people are a central resource and perform better when treated well.
5 Hands on, value driven approach, that is, values are important, not just a search for profit.
6 They do not diversify outside their range of central expertise.
7 A simple form, lean staff, a non-complex management structure that can be understood easily, and no large corporate staff.
8 Simultaneous tight–loose properties, the coexistence of tight central direction and maximum personal autonomy. The central control is achieved through value systems, and through painstaking attention to detail.

Peters and Waterman (1982) argue that people matter to business, and should not be neglected, as either workers or customers; that workplace culture is as important as quantitative data in managing a workforce; and that innovation is crucial to companies and will only be obtained if they protect their creative people, allowing them autonomy, and decentralise their decision making. In short, people need to be motivated to work; if a company can do this it will be successful; the way to do it is to treat employees positively as creative human beings.

Management theory originating from both Taylor and Peters tends to assume that the theory is relevant to the coordination of all types of workers. However, the variety of circumstances is such that this universal approach is problematic. A third view, taken by writers such as Handy (1984, 1990) and Atkinson (1986), suggests that different segments of the workforce are, and should be, managed differently. Atkinson suggests a duality of core and periphery, while Handy suggests a three-fold division for which he uses the metaphor of the shamrock leaf.

Atkinson (1986) argues that there is a developing division within many companies between a core and a peripheral workforce. The core is managed by attempting to gain the workers' commitment, in a way which parallels much of new wave management thinking. These workers are given secure contracts and high wages; their jobs are enriched and diversified; they are encouraged to be functionally flexible and to extend the range of tasks they are prepared to perform. In contrast, workers in the periphery are managed more severely, in ways which have some similarities with Taylorism (though some crucial differences too). They are on insecure contracts and low wages. They are numerically flexible, in that the number of hours they work may be easily varied by the use of part-time contracts, or temporary contracts. They are often distanced from the main employer by a mediated relationship through a sub-contractor.

Handy's (1990) account includes these two groups which he describes in similar terms, but he also adds a third group, suggesting a division similar to that of the three leaves of a shamrock. This third leaf is that of workers who are sub-contracted out. Thus his model is more complex, effectively splitting Atkinson's periphery into two. While the sub-contracted workforce has less good conditions than the core, there remains a question as to whether those who are sub-contracted have good or poor rates of pay. Hakim's work on homeworking (1987a,b), which suggests that a significant section of these workers is well paid and highly skilled, appears to support this more differentiated model.

While the core, functionally flexible workers have much in common with the forms of work relations described and advocated by new wave management theorists such as Peters, the coincidence of the periphery with Taylorist practices is less clear. Under Taylorist management workers had regular jobs, working regular hours on relatively secure contracts, even though the power to hire and fire was regarded as part of the managerial prerogative. The extent of the insecurity of the new employment relations in the periphery goes beyond conventional Taylorist practice, while the distancing from the main employer involved in sub-contracting is likewise outside conventional Taylorist conceptions of management.

Is it possible to apply new wave management theory, such as that of Peters and Waterman, to all work settings, or is it contextually specific? Is it possible to apply it to a public sector service? In particular, is it possible to apply it to forms of work where performance is difficult to monitor? While identifying the differences from the traditional Taylorist approach, Wood (1989) is critical of the new wave management literature for two main reasons. First, it under-estimates the significance of politics and power within organisations. Secondly, it has an inadequate empirical base in that it draws upon a restricted range of examples.

Is public sector management different from private sector management? Flynn (1990) argues that there are two main differences in that there is no profit motive and there is no competition – in short, a lack of basic market features. There are other principles, however, such as equitable treatment and allocation of resources according to need. These lead to different concepts and ways of measuring success: sales and profits are not the issue, in public services the attraction of customers is rarely a problem, investment decisions are not set to maximise profits. However, the absence of a profit motive is not in itself a barrier to competition. Bartlett and LeGrand (1994) suggest that the 'not for profit' health care organisations in the USA provide a theoretical model for NHS Trusts. They note the possibility that Trusts may evolve as 'labour managed', that is, run in such a way as to give maximum weight to the decisions that benefit dominant members of the workforce and board. Such a model requires a unity of purpose between senior clinicians, senior management, and board members, and embodies a risk that salary increases to senior staff, or the payment of over-generous job related perks, become a significant motivational aim.

What is the relevance of these ideas to the health professionals under consideration here? The first issue is whether and, if so where, professional workers fit within these models. We shall argue that the professions share many crucial characteristics with the prescriptions of new wave management theorists, although some are missing. The second issue is the utility of the models for understanding the issues and dilemmas of the fragmentation of work relations which we described in Chapter 4. Both approaches to management have engaged with the problem of coordinating labour processes which are fragmented in order to manage them efficiently. They contain theoretical accounts as to how these dilemmas appear and are contained. We will explore these below in order to understand the fragmentation described in Chapter 4.

Medicine and new wave management

There are many ways in which the old professions, especially medicine, appear to be good examples of new wave management practice. Traditional professionals display high motivation and commitment to their work. They are highly trained and value this training. They are self-monitoring and regulating. They are highly autonomous and have very little direct supervision. They have high levels of functional flexibility, and flexible time working. They have a high level of commitment to the customer, in so far as this is the patient. There is a strong professional culture which supports high standards of work and commitment. Indeed, the account that medicine produces of itself is quite close to the new wave manager's ideal worker.

The eight key points of Peters and Waterman's (1982) account are closely reflected in medicine. The first principle was a bias for action and eagerness to experiment. Doctors are engaged in active, continuous monitoring and modification of treatment plans, and experimentation is the basis of their claim to scientific knowledge. The second principle was that of being close to the consumer. In so far as the consumer is considered to be the patient, then doctors are very close to their customers, being engaged in a direct relationship with them. The Hippocratic oath, which is the centre of the doctor's code of ethics, puts concern for the patient above all other concerns. The third was worker autonomy. Clinical freedom is a cherished medical principle. Consultants have considerable freedom of action in their decisions as to how the patient is to be treated and considerable discretion over the organisation of their own work. The fourth principle was that productivity comes through people. Medical personnel are highly trained with longer periods of training (in universities and junior hospital positions) than most other workers. The fifth is that values are important in the goals of a company, not merely profit. A commitment to the value of patient health is a major hallmark of the NHS. The aim to restore health, and to provide this regardless of ability to pay, are key elements of the NHS culture. The sixth of specialisation is clearly present. The seventh, of a simple form of management, is present if the focus is kept within medicine which has a hierarchy based on a consultant-led team or firm. The eighth of simultaneous tight–loose properties, of central value systems and personal autonomy is again present in medicine.

There are, however, some important points where divergence between the professional and new wave management practice might be identified. The first major qualification is over the principle of closeness to the customer. If the patient is the customer then there is not an issue. However, it is not clear that the new organisation of the NHS since 1989 constructs the patient as the customer, since the patient is not a 'purchaser'. In the new markets there are several contenders for the title of customer. The purchasers of the hospital doctor's services are the health authority and GP fund holders. The third principle of autonomy does not apply so clearly for doctors beneath the level of consultant. Medicine has a very strong internal hierarchy in which the positions of house officer, senior house officer, and registrar are described as training grades, thus not entitling the holder to the same degree of autonomy. Further qualifications on the principle of medical autonomy were found with the relationship between junior doctors and senior nurses on the ward, described in Chapter 2. The seventh principle of a lean, clear management structure is also problematic, with the increasing significance of general managers, since the Griffiths Report (NHS Management Enquiry, 1983), and the increasing complexity of financial structures, since *Working for Patients* (Department of Health, 1989a).

Most of these caveats relate to the position of junior hospital doctors. They not only have their decision making circumscribed by others, they are on different kinds of contracts. In some ways junior doctors are more like the third leaf of Handy's shamrock, than either core or periphery. Junior doctors are on temporary contracts, until they reach consultant grade. While all grades of doctors beneath that of consultant are called training grades, these are also the main work grades of the profession. Despite these various caveats, the parallels between the management of medicine and new wave management are striking.

We see a process of change in medicine, from a pre-Fordist system of professional autonomy up to 1985, followed by a move in a Fordist direction with the introduction of general management principles in the mid 1980s. The second change followed a new wave management approach, with the development of an internal market and the formation of Trusts in 1991–92, but with the retention of a very large degree of central control, and the continuation of Taylorist management at a unit level. Since then the evidence is of a sharply contested divide between proponents of a more forceful extension of human resource management (Seccombe and Buchan, 1994), and an increasingly articulated desire for 'a reassertion of the old values relating to staff' (*Health Service Management Journal*, March 1994: 3). A third set of changes arise from the need to address the issue of junior doctors' hours.

While the current changes in the NHS are the main interest here, nevertheless an exclusive focus on contemporary issues obscures the radical nature of the 1985 Griffiths change from a pre-Fordist service dominated by the health professions, notably medicine, to an organisational structure led by general managers. We share the opinion of Seccombe and Buchan (1994: 181) that the Griffiths' reforms 'provided the structural changes necessary to enable the organisational and cultural changes implicit in the reforms of the 1990s [to take place]'. The next section therefore examines the introduction of general management, before considering the impact of internal markets, and the changing hours of junior doctors.

General management   The introduction of general management following the Griffiths Report (NHS Management Enquiry, 1983) was designed to create greater efficiency by increasing the capacity for decisive leadership. The new general managers at unit (hospital) and district level were expected to take decisions previously taken by negotiation and consensus among professional groups. It was intended to reduce the autonomy of disparate professional and occupational groups and subject them to a common authority. It tried to develop a tighter line of management up to the Health Minister, with a clear remit over the management of resources. Workers with the title of manager were introduced amid much controversy. Nevertheless, one of the changes of the past decade has been the growing importance of the idea that there should be more management in order to produce effective work, in opposition to practices which are accused of letting things drift and in which work is said to be organised by workers for workers, rather than for customers. In particular, it has been suggested that workers had captured the welfare state and the nationalised industries so that they were run for the workers, rather than for the consumer and the public. Managers were introduced in the mid-1980s, followed by markets in the early 1990s, apparently in order to change this, so that the industry or service was run for the public as consumer. The rival claim is that the workers, especially the professional workers, were doing a good job, and the government's interest in intervention is merely to cut or contain the cost of the welfare state (Harrison et al., 1992; Owens and Glennerster, 1990; Strong and Robinson, 1990).

Flynn (1992) argues that the introduction of general management shifted the form of regulation in the NHS, introducing a number of forms of control. He suggests that the recent changes in the health service have altered the balance of power between the doctors and the administrators-turned-managers so that the former group has lost power to the latter.

> An unprecedented battery of measures and techniques for audit, evaluation, monitoring and surveillance now exist. These constitute the principal devices through which the structure of control in health is accomplished . . . Medical autonomy has been increasingly circumscribed by the extension of bureaucratic and managerial authority. Professional prerogatives and technical discretion are no longer taken for granted: accountability is more than ever defined in terms of corporate objectives, defined, translated and enforced by state-appointed executives. (Flynn, 1992: 183)

However, Kerrison, Packwood and Buxton (1994) provide evidence that contradicts Flynn's belief that medical audit represents an increase in managerial influence over the medical profession. Instead, they depict medical audit as being predominantly a process whereby junior medical staff can anticipate the clinical preferences of consultants, and a symbolic proof of clinicians' commitment and vocation. Their comments fit in with the scepticism expressed by Owens and Glennerster about the impact of management change, which is discussed below. There are some aspects of the introduction of general management which share features with new wave management, in particular the focus on building a new culture within the NHS. The new general managers constitute a social group within the NHS which is committed to the implementation of a new way of running the health service. It is not simply a matter of government ministers announcing changes; there is a social constituency with its own agenda and culture and some considerable power. Indeed, we might almost refer to this as a new social movement, given the shape this initiative has taken (see Clarke and Newman, 1994; Strong and Robinson, 1990).

There is no doubt that considerable managerial zeal was created in the mid and late 1980s to reform the NHS. The feeling of a new wave of management made it appear almost a social movement among managers who were being inspired to do better. It started with a focus on locating decision making lower down so as to encourage more worker responsibility, in classic new wave management style. However, there were two ways in which it failed to complete its 'mission'. First, the full agenda was restricted by the context of fierce cost containment, curtailing the new wave agenda of developing employees' potential. Secondly, there was no market, a feature which Peters and Waterman (1982) took as a prerequisite. The process of creating one met with difficulties derived from the problems of measuring performance.

However, not everyone is convinced that general management did achieve the changes it was billed as creating. While most analysts agree that the intention behind the introduction of general management was to create a stronger line of management, some, such as Owens and Glennerster (1990), are more circumspect as to whether the introduction of general management in itself had quite the impact that both its friends and foes attributed to it, while recognising that it was a significant symbolic change. They are thus sceptical that anything has significantly changed with the introduction of general management: the real power relations have not significantly shifted. Porters, cleaners and clerical staff have an organiser external to their unit, and doctors are 'outside the system of accountability at the sub-unit level', with consultants' contracts in many districts being held at regional level. They suggest that the 'structural changes were more apparent than real, as they did not signify changed power relationships' (Owens and Glennerster, 1990: 111). The informants in our own study echoed some of the scepticism. With the hindsight of almost a decade we suggest that their scepticism is misplaced, and that the significance of the introduction of general management into the NHS lay in providing a structural basis for the introduction of an internal market and a re-invigorated form of Taylorism.

The impact of a health market   Quite apart from the nature of health service management, the existence of a market in health care in itself requires changes in the working practice of doctors. The management of markets is discussed in Chapter 6; here we note the impact on the working practices of NHS doctors.

The existence of service contracts obliges medical staff to ensure that payment has been secured before commencing the treatment of non-emergency patients. Before markets were introduced it was recognised that an obligation to check on payment would be contrary to the culture and ethos of medicine as it has been practiced in the NHS since its inception. Equally, accepting a particular patient for admission in preference to another for funding reasons is also wholly alien to the concept of equitable access to care. While this has never been an achievable target, as admission rates and waiting list comparisons between regions and districts show, the aim of equitable access has been present throughout the existence of the NHS. Giving priority for admissions to patients whose funding is secure, in preference to those with uncertain funding requires adjustments to medical practice that challenge the value system of the profession. Mumford (1993: 4, 5) began an account of managing staff in hospitals with the phrase 'We are heading into a period of gritty realism'. He then commented:

> Balancing business practices with those of a public service is an increasingly taxing demand upon hospitals . . . Now we are in a position where individuals, professional groups, and whole hospitals are acting at the very edge, if not outside of, their own value bases. Witness the struggle with the two-tier system for GP fundholders, 'overperforming' hospitals, or the preferential treatment given to patients coming in on extra-contractual referrals . . . If you put this together with the erosion of the NHS as a reasonably secure employer, the pressure on hospital staff is building.

Junior doctors' hours   Quite apart from questions as to the governance of the NHS, or the impact of markets, there are also dilemmas for the management of medicine that arise from the changes needed to deal with the problem of reducing the excessively long hours of the junior doctors. The response to this problem has sometimes involved a move away from the traditional model. Junior house officers and senior house officers work the longest hours. The traditional view within medicine is to see these long hours as part of a historic custom, and as an inevitable short phase in the life of a young doctor.

Junior doctors' hours are widely regarded as excessive, not only by junior doctors themselves, but the government, which has set up a 'new deal' for doctors (NHS Management Executive, 1991), and also nurse leaders. One senior nurse leader and member of one of nursing's leading bodies made the following comment on the working hours of doctors, calling for a form of time management more akin to that of nursing:

> *Senior nurse leader*: The system they work is totally antiquated and barbaric and if they actually put their own house in order a lot of this problem [of doctors being woken at night by nursing demands] wouldn't arise – like proper shift working. To expect people to be on call for a whole weekend is just idiotic.

There are current efforts to reduce the number of hours of junior doctors. However, while this senior nurse saw shift working as the solution, this is not the remedy advanced by other bodies. The proposal from the SCOPME (1991) Report, following on from the NHS Management Executive report *Junior Doctors: the New Deal* (1991), suggested that some tasks of junior doctors could go to nurses (simple suturing; administration of intravenous drugs; 'topping up' of epidurals), while others could go to technical, clerical and administrative staff (locating empty beds; delivering requests and obtaining results of laboratory tests; portering duties; routine blood taking; filing results in case notes). So while the nurse quoted above would deal with the over-working of junior doctors by suggesting a traditional form of time management via shift working within medicine, that of SCOPME was to re-draw the boundary between medicine and other occupations.

Nursing and new wave management

Nursing has a different relationship to new wave management practice from medicine. Its existing practice is further away, though some of the aspirations of current nurse leaders are quite close. Nurses lack the important characteristics of autonomy of decision making which is such a key feature of new wave management. Thus in comparison to medicine, nurses are much less organised along new wave management principles. The first principle of a bias for action and eagerness to experiment is lacking since nurses are considerably rule bound, needing to follow detailed procedures. The second characteristic, being close to the consumer, is present, in so far as the patient is constructed as the consumer. The third, autonomy, is significantly less present than it is for doctors, though this varies according to the mode of ward organisation. Nurses are highly trained, so the fourth principle is present, though whether they are considered to be well treated is a matter of debate. Nurses are as value driven as doctors, with key professional goals promoting the welfare of patients (though, of course, as with medicine, varyingly endorsed in practice). They have a simple form of management within nursing itself, but a highly complex one if their relationship with medicine, general management and ancillary staff is included. Overall, the eighth principle of 'tight–loose' properties is lacking because of the lack of personal autonomy, leaving only the tight central direction. There are, though, indications of change. The recent development of primary nursing is evidence of a move towards a looser style of professional governance. The decision by the UKCC to end the system of extended role certification is further evidence of the emergence of a different culture within some sections of the profession. Primary nursing has elements that are compatible with new wave management principles.

Traditionally, nursing has often been considered not to be a fully developed profession. The control over their work by others, especially doctors, the rule-bound internal hierarchy, and the lack of control over the client who 'belongs' to the consultant are three of the features which preclude this. These are basically the same features as those which distance nursing from new wave management.

So where do nurses fit? Are they organised along Taylorist principles of management? Are they core workers or peripheral workers as in Atkinson's model, or the second or third leaf of Handy's shamrock? Are they about to suffer the collapse of the conventional career and move from core to periphery as suggested by Davies (1990) and McSweeney (1991)? They do not fit any of the models very well.

Nurses are currently closest in organisation to the Taylorist model, though the development of primary nursing is different, emphasising a greater degree of autonomy in decision making. Nursing is rule bound and relatively closely monitored by a conventional system of line management, but departs from a Taylorist model in being highly trained and skilled. They are core and essential staff so also fit the core of both Atkinson and Handy's models. However, Davies (1990) and McSweeney (1991) argue that this may be changing as more nurses take on work part-time and interrupt careers to have children. Nurses as a whole do not fit the model of the new periphery, as described by either Atkinson or Handy, in that the majority of trained nurses have secure contracts of employment. While some nurses will be on temporary contracts as agency nurses, possibly for only a few days, or as bank nurses who negotiate intermittent work with the hospital, and a few have fixed term contracts or work as part-timers, the majority still have conventional permanent contracts, though the movement of budgets to ward level is seen as encouraging the ward sister to be more 'flexible' in the employment of nursing staff. The Audit Commission note this with evident approval:

> One NHS hospital in the Audit Commission sample is well on the way toward devolved budgets. Ward sisters control the pay budgets and are responsible for the costs of bank and agency staff. As a result, the sisters have started to cancel temporary staff when the workload does not justify their employment, and buy them in when it does. (Audit Commission, 1991: 53)

Nursing is changing rapidly. Registered nurses (RNs) form a more highly trained elite, with another group of less trained, less well paid nursing assistants. Project 2000 is a central part of this strategy, upgrading the training of the qualified nurses, but creating a need for a new grade of staff to replace the work of student nurses, now college based and not part of the hospital staffing establishment. The new staff are health care assistants, who have only six months' training, leading to NVQs up to level 3. Registered nurses control their training and assess their work, and they work under the direction of registered nurses. Health care assistants will have considerably lower wages, and these may be regionally variable (Chapman, 1991). A pattern where some but not all nurses become part of the periphery is already occurring, although it is not yet widespread.

So, is nursing an anomaly? Or are the theories of the changes in the management of employment wrong? If we take health work as a whole, we can see the introduction of the kinds of insecure and temporary contracts Atkinson and Handy predict, but they are found more among the ancillary staff than trained nurses, although they are predicted to develop here (Davies, 1990). The position of bank and agency nurses is as yet somewhat anomalous, in that the insecurity of agency work has to be balanced by the higher salary paid, and bank nursing offers valued flexibility to the nurse as well as to the hospital. Curiously, junior doctors have always had temporary contracts and uncertain hours but with clearly specified duties in a manner similar to that of Handy's highly skilled temporary workers.

But workers as highly skilled as nurses are not usually so closely managed as nurses. There are several groups of highly skilled largely female occupations which fit uneasily into the standard division of the workforce into core and periphery, or primary and secondary. Nursing like teaching, social work, librarianship and some secretarial and administrative work is skilled work which is not usually included in the core or elite (Walby, 1989). Is it that workers with this level of skill have typically managed to gain more autonomy, but that when they are female workers, they have lacked the political power to make these claims stick in the wider social arena, especially where state endorsement is needed? That is, is the lack of professional autonomy of nursing due to the position of women in a patriarchal society (see Witz, 1992)? Or is this the face of things to come, as the current political initiative seeks to contain professional power, especially that bound up in the welfare state? Elston (1991) has argued that we are seeing a slight decline in the professional power of medicine. Coburn (1988) has shown that Canadian nurses similarly display this mix of high skill and low autonomy and control, so these processes are not unique to the UK.

The challenge of measuring performance outcomes and staffing needs is a long-standing issue in nursing management. There have been attempts to develop formulas by which nurse managers may more accurately determine how many nurses are needed in a ward with a particular number of patients with different levels of dependency and need for nursing. For instance, the North West Region pioneered a project to determine this called 'Teamwork', based on their research on previous models (Bagust et al., 1988) complete with its own newsletter, *Teamwork*, software experts and demonstration days. 'Teamwork' may initially sound like a Taylorist practice, but the fact that the system operates within nursing suggests caution in describing it simply as a management tool. In particular, the careful adjustment of the type and amount of nursing to the particular situation on a ward at a given moment, rather than a standard number of nurses rigorously adhered to whatever the actual circumstances, means that this development is more in keeping with the customised packages of care for the consumer of new wave management, than that of Taylorism.

There is considerable debate as to the extent to which nursing can be enhanced by improved management, by increasing the skill level of nurses, or simply by employing more 'pairs of hands'. The Audit Commission (1991: 8) suggests that 'there is considerable scope to enhance the quality of nursing within existing resource constraints'. The Commission suggests a series of changes in ward and hospital management of nurses for implementation by nursing management to achieve this.

Carr-Hill et al. (1992) suggest that improving the skill level of nursing would make a significant difference to the outcome for patients. They attempt to assess the impact of skill on nursing care, taking great care to develop effective instruments to do this in a context of a concern to measure nursing outcomes as well as nursing process. Using a modified version of 'Qualpacs', an assessment tool for measuring the quality of nursing care given to patients (Wandelt and Ager, 1974), they conclude that the standard of nursing care is significantly increased by employing higher grade staff. They show that this is a robust finding in a number of ways. It is complicated by being affected by the mix of nursing skills, in that the quality of higher grade staff is pulled down by the presence of lower grade staff, though that of the latter is improved. The study finally assesses the cost implications of increasing the training of staff, although the comparison with increasing the numbers of less skilled staff is far from clear in the report. An increase of staffing by one grade costs 15 per cent of the salary bill and produces a 6 per cent increase in effective range of Qualpac ratings. 'The overall conclusions therefore of this study are simple: investment in employing qualified staff, providing post qualification training and developing effective methods of organising nursing care appeared to pay dividends in the delivery of good quality patient care' (Carr-Hill et al., 1992: 144).

Not surprisingly, this report was welcomed by the unions associated with nursing, as supporting a strategy of upskilling for nursing, as indicated by the following comment by the national health secretary of the National Union of Public Employees, Malcolm Wing: 'We have waited for this report for a long time and hope it will bury the lie being peddled by some of the NHS management executive that there is no relationship between quality of care and a well-qualified workforce' (*Guardian* 21 October 1992). These changes are those at the upper end of nursing, where the focus is on improving nursing's already considerable system of qualifications. There is also a significant boundary for nursing with the new NVQ certified health workers. These assistants may perform tasks that nursing either does not want to do or which managers will insist on giving to these cheaper workers. As nursing upgrades there is the possibility that the newly empowered managers will energetically seek out cheaper workers.

Fragmentation and theories of the management of work

Chapter 4 identified several sources of tension between medicine and nursing which stemmed from the fragmentation of the ward and the doctor–nurse team. In so far as there is specialisation of work, yet a common product, then there is necessarily the need to both specialise and reintegrate. In the case of health work this is clear: the consultant's tasks are separate from those of the nurse and the house officer, in order to realise the efficiencies of specialisation of training and expertise, and of less paid workers doing some tasks to save the time of more highly paid workers. Yet it is essential to reintegrate their tasks since the patient is common to both, and to reintegrate the budget for their services because contracts are for services provided by the directorate not for the work of single professions.

The ways and degrees to which this is done are present in the different theories of the management of employment. Traditional Taylorist conceptions of work separated the conception of the job from its execution. The tasks were reintegrated using a clear hierarchy of management, but this integration is a challenge because management and workers would each prefer to maintain their knowledge of the conception, in order better to control the labour process and its rewards. Under new wave management, specialisation is often reconceptualised as decentralisation and as important in the process of locating the producer close enough to consumers to be responsive to their desires. Reintegration is to be achieved through a strong common value system. New wave management thus fragments through decentralisation and the market, and reintegrates through culture.

In the working lives of our doctors and nurses there was considerable fragmentation of their team in the name of efficiency. This was illustrated in the examples, described in earlier chapters, of communication failure, tasks not done as and when wanted, outlier patients and multi-consultant wards, and when doctor–doctor conflict affected treatment. Reintegration was attempted by tactics such as bleeps, which themselves could generate considerable friction, and strategies such as the introduction of general management.

Underlying these sources of fragmentation and attempts at reintegration are different theories of management, as well as the interests of different groups. General management represents a Taylorist intervention to reintegrate a health service which was considered to have diverged too far from the interests of the consumer and to have constituent groups which were insufficiently integrated to take the necessary strategic decisions. The introduction of internal markets was supposed to reintegrate the producer with the concerns of the consumer, by using the market to compel a new focus on the users of services.

Nurses and management

While most accounts of management in the NHS presume they are dealing with two groups – doctors and managers – they should be dealing also with a third large group: nurses. The omission of nurses is more than an oversight and is a serious flaw, partly because nurses consume so large a proportion of the NHS budget. The omission of this large female occupation from the management hierarchy is itself a source of struggle.

Nurse representatives have sometimes been included in the senior management committees of the NHS and sometimes excluded. As Table 5.1 shows, the high point of nurse representation was in the aftermath of the 1974 and 1982 reorganisation when nurses as well as doctors obtained a statutory right for a reserved place on the area health authorities, area team of officers, district management team (in 1974) and the district health authority and district management team (in 1982). The Griffiths changes implemented in 1985 removed automatic representation of nurses from the district management team, while retaining a place for public health doctors. This

Table 5.1   *Statutory representation of doctors and nurses on NHS Boards: England and Wales*[1]

1948[2]

	Hospital management committees (non-teaching)	Hospital boards of governors (teaching)	Local health authorities
Doctors	Y	Y	Y
Nurses	N	N	N

1974[3]

	Area health authorities	Area team of officers	District management team
Doctors	Y	Y: 1/4	Y: 3/6
Nurses	Y	Y: 1/4	Y: 1/6

1982[4]

	District health authority	District management team
Doctors	Y	Y: 3/6
Nurses	Y	Y: 1/6

1985 (Griffiths management structure implemented)[5]

	District health authority	District management team
Doctors	Y	Y: 1/6
Nurses	Y	N

1991 (*Working for Patients* Reforms)[6]

	District health authorities		NHS Trust Boards	
	5 Non-exec. directors	5 exec. directors	5 non-exec. directors	5 exec. directors
Doctors	N	N	N	Y: 1/5
Nurses	N	N	N	Y: 1/5

'Y' indicates that there is at least one place on the board or team reserved for a medical/nursing representative. 'N' indicates that there is no statutory obligation to reserve a place for a doctor/nurse. Figures refer to the ratio of reserved places for each profession.

[1] The organisation of the NHS in Scotland is different from the English and Welsh structure. Levitt and Wall (1992) give a concise outline of the Scottish pattern.

[2] NHS Act of 1946 was implemented in 1948, establishing the NHS.

[3] The NHS was reorganised in 1974, following the 1972 National Health Service Reorganisation Bill. Area health authorities were established.

[4] A further reorganisation followed in 1982, abolishing the area health authorities,

and establishing district health authorities. These changes were set out in the circular HC(80)8 *Health Services Development: Structure and Management*, 1980.

[5] In 1984–85 health authorities began to implement the proposals initiated by the NHS Management Enquiry, chaired by Sir Roy Griffiths, and confirmed in Circular HC(84)13 [45] *Health Service Management: Implementation of the NHS Management Enquiry*. Before the 1984–85 changes the composition of the management team was laid down by statute. Following this restructuring, the district general manager, with the approval of the health authority, could select the management team. Some chose to keep a nurse on the team. The community physician had to be a member of the management team.

[6] The 1989 White Paper *Working for Patients* recommended radical changes in NHS organisation, which were enacted in the 1990 National Health Service and Community Care Act and implemented in the NHS in April 1991. This included proposals to form NHS Trusts, and established smaller Health Authorities, modelled on the lines of a commercial board, with executive and non-executive Directors. Non-executive directors are appointed on a personal basis, with no statutory representation for medical or nursing staff. As in 1984, the chief executive of a health authority chooses the executive directors following consultation with the non-executive directors. A public health consultant is usually one of the executive members of the health authority, though there was no statutory requirement for either a medical or nursing executive appointment in the 1990 Act. Of the executive directors only the chief executive and the director of finance have statutory appointments as executive directors.

Unlike Health Authorities, NHS Trust Board executive directors have to include a doctor and a nurse.

generated much controversy among nurses. An automatic place for nurses on the NHS Trust Boards was created in the 1991 changes.

The extent of control and influence of the nursing profession as represented by senior nurses over the direction of health service policy has changed over time. Robinson (1992) also suggests that January 1985 was a low point in nursing's importance for public policy. This was a consequence of the implementation of the Griffiths Report with the introduction of general management into the NHS. She describes reports of chief nursing officers at district and regional levels of the health service losing their jobs, losing control over the nursing budget, and losing line management control over nursing. In response, in spring 1986 the Royal College of Nursing launched a major campaign in the national press. One of the advertisements asked whether 'the general manager knows his coccyx from his humerus?' However, Robinson (1992: 1) suggests that the campaign was almost completely unsuccessful in resisting these changes in the management of nursing.

Robinson addresses the lack of interest in nursing policy issues, and this despite the size of the workforce – half a million. This lack of interest she labels 'the black hole theory of nursing'. While the Griffiths reforms were certainly intended to control medicine, nursing was merely 'caught in the cross-fire'. One of the reasons identified for this 'black hole' has been the historic lack of critical well-educated nurses, but the different interests of health workers have also been seen as significant: 'Nurses were the members of staff who most often raised questions of equity and humanity in health care. Financial matters preoccupied most of the managers' (Robinson, 1992: 5). Robinson has some highly critical points which highlight current problems of the 'black hole' of policy making for nursing:

1 Nurses are virtually never involved in concrete policy decision making processes; what may pass as a nursing decision is in reality acquiescence to others' prior formulations.

2 Issues that primarily concern nurses (for example, maintaining adequate staffing levels in order to ensure humane and equitable standards of care) are either kept off the formal policy agenda or disguised as nurses' inability to manage scarce resources adequately.

3 Contemporary health policy initiatives seek to control the apparently limitless power of medicine to expand by bringing in cost-containment policies which set nurse against nurse . . . Whilst for some nurses cost-containment measures provide an opportunity for enhancing their professional power and status, for others, the result is increased workload and an impoverishment of both their working conditions and their ability to deliver high standards of nursing care. For yet others, such policies jeopardise their very jobs. The 'order to care in a society that refuses to value caring' (Reverby 1987) results in conflicts which extend across the qualified/unqualified, waged/ unwaged female caring divides. (Robinson, 1992: 8)

The Report of the Audit Commission (1991) on nurse managers gives a clear impression of how nursing issues are moving from a peripheral place in a hospital's agenda to a more central role, but makes it clear that this process is disjointed and reactive, with only one of the ten hospitals studied having a clear nursing strategy.

Nursing is too important a component of patient care and consumes and controls too large a proportion of hospital resources, to be left to develop in isolation or as an afterthought to clinical reorganisation. The commit-ment of the whole of the hospital and unit management team to a common vision of the way nursing should develop is necessary for improvements in patient care and effective use of nurses. The best way to achieve this commitment is for nurses to take the lead and, with general managers and clinicians, jointly to develop a comprehensive nursing strategy. (Audit Commission, 1991: 57)

Our interest is in the role of these general managers in inter-professional relations. There are two issues here: whether they introduced competing lines of authority which significantly changed the organisation of professional work (Glennerster et al., 1986;

Owens and Glennerster, 1990); secondly, their role in the areas of disagreement between the professions that we uncovered in our study. Differences in the management of medicine and nursing were sometimes at the root of difficulties in interprofessional working. How far are general managers involved in settling interprofessional disputes, and establishing cultural values within hospitals that transcend some of the variations between professions?

Discrepant lines of authority?

The fragmentation of the organisation of medicine and nursing has a number of dimensions. One recent addition to both the problem and the solution to these has been the introduction of general management. General management was intended to increase the degree of cohesion by producing one superior line of authority. However, some commentators have discussed whether this has simply added another layer of competing authority (Glennerster et al., 1986; Owens and Glennerster, 1990; Strong and Robinson, 1990). This was the initial view of Glennerster and colleagues in their study (1986) of the impact of general management on nursing; a view which they modified by the time the research project was completed (Owens and Glennerster, 1990). A not dissimilar ambivalence was expressed by Strong and Robinson (1990) in their discussion of the introduction of general management into NHS hospitals.

Glennerster et al. (1986) discuss the impact the introduction of general management might have on nurses as a result of introducing discrepant lines of accountability with both a professional line through nursing and another through general management. In the previous, Salmon-inspired, managerial system nurses had their own professional hierarchy which was the basis of their accountability. Under the Griffiths-inspired changes, general managers took the top places in this system. Nurses were not included as nurses in the top reaches of management and few nurses were appointed to the general management posts, though subsequently nurses have moved into general management at various levels. In the interim report on their research Glennerster and colleagues (1986) stressed the difficulties which they saw arising from the problem of dual accountability for nurses to the professional nursing hierarchy on the one hand and to the general management structure on the other. What would happen if there were conflicts between these two chains of accountability? Nurses reported that they were uneasy about which line of command they should follow if there were conflicts and how they would make a decision as to which they would follow.

This was in contrast to the Salmon-based management structure in which there was a single chain of command for nurses. This was considered to be a very serious defect of the general management system. It was expected that conflict and misunderstandings would arise.

In their later work at the end of the project, Owens and Glennerster (1990) suggest that this tension was not the serious problem they had initially thought. They found that such issues did not occur on a daily basis, though when they did occur they had the potential to be serious. They state that potential problems are avoided and that a series of practices had developed to resolve potential difficulties. One of the ways that this was done was by appointing nurses to the positions of general management in those units where nurses were the majority of the workforce. Sensitive individual solutions were found by others.

There was initial uncertainty as to the extent of the responsibility of the senior nurse and the unit managers, but by the end of their research period the interconnections were realised and both professionals and managers understood that the other would need to be involved. Thus the early suggestions that these changes would give rise to chronic problems of dual accountability were discovered to be unfounded as a result of the management system adapting by more regularly including senior nurses, by the sensitive handling of points of conflict by senior nurses, and by the development of management practices which recognised the impossibility of separating professional and managerial issues.

Strong and Robinson (1990) describe the introduction of general management as an attempt to solve the stasis engendered by the fragmentation of authority into competing groups of workers. It was initially seen as a kind of crusade in which the new managers saw their new jobs as an important opportunity to improve the NHS.

The stultifying effect of a bureaucratic organisation run by administrators was to be replaced with a thrusting new world of dynamic entrepreneurial managers. But Strong and Robinson are fully aware of the contrary model, in which the NHS is an organisation which is, by international standards, extremely cheap for the level of health care delivered.

Strong and Robinson consider several problems in the management of doctors and nurses which are often a mirror image of each other. Doctors are considered to be too individualistic, paying little attention to the interests of others in the health service. There could be fierce competition between doctors for resources, but they would close ranks against outsiders. The old health administrators were considered to have simply given in to this medical syndicalism.

Nurses were considered to suffer from the opposite fault: to be too deferential, and to be too accepting of a bureaucratic chain of command.

> There was, then, a quite extraordinary contrast in managers' eyes between the individual power of doctors and the collective feebleness of nurses; between medicine's influence at the highest levels and nursing's notional representation; between doctors' fierce syndicalism and nursing's massive internal hierarchy . . . Nursing's hierarchy stemmed not so much from within nursing itself, as from the many powerful forces – medicine, gender and the demands of an extremely labour-intensive industry – which had created, shaped and controlled the nursing trade . . . Doctors would not be led. Nurses did not know how to lead . . . Too many nurse managers were defensive, sectarian, isolationist, Luddite. Too many doctors dropped in on the chairman, rang the treasurer at breakfast, burst in through the administrator's door and answered only to God . . . (Strong and Robinson, 1990: 39, 65–6)

However, there is a remaining question as to whether general managers introduced a single line of command or merely added another line of accountability. From one perspective it was simply hubris for the general managers to believe that they constituted the main integrative force. General managers themselves constitute a special interest group – they are as much a tribe as any other group of health workers. They were a new specialism, though one with greater ability to claim the label of general than other groups, though this could be contested, especially by consultants who also consider that they represent the general good.

General managers in our study

The general managers in the five hospitals in our study had widely different practices in relation to interprofessional disputes. When asked about interprofessional conflict, our unit general managers typically did not spontaneously mention the issues we had discovered in our study. However, when asked whether specific issues had been considered, they usually indicated that the matter had indeed been addressed within their unit. Some tensions were contained at a low level, while others came more insistently before their attention. An issue which would be left to be resolved at a clinical level in some units would in others have received intervention from the unit general manager. Some unit general managers dealt with these tensions in an *ad hoc* manner as the occasion demanded, sometimes with a task force to deal with it. Others had set up standing committees specifically to deal with an itemised list of interprofessional issues. These special committees themselves varied as to whether they were composed of both professions and management, or both the professions, or were doctor led. In short, there was little pattern to the extent and manner in which unit general managers engaged with issues of interprofessional tensions and conflicts, but they recognised the list of issues that we presented to them.

There are some national initiatives to which unit general managers sometimes make specific responses, for example, that of reducing the excessively long hours of junior doctors. One of our unit general managers chaired the local group attempting to implement the reduction in hours and, when asked if they ever intervened in interprofessional disputes, made this the main issue about which a response was given:

> *Unit general manager*: We are relatively well staffed, which I think is a great help . . . I'm actually currently chairing the local implementation group, which is the junior doctors' hours group . . . under the junior doctors' hours arrangements we've been asked to look at the work which the nurses do to see if they could do more, to relieve some of the work of the junior doctors. Now, that is an issue in that context . . . where the doctors feel that the nurses could do things like drips . . . One issue that's just blowing up is prescribing of aspirin and over-the-counter drugs and where the nursing administration has said 'No, thou shalt not do that.'

Tensions between doctors and nurses were regarded as inevitable by most of our unit general managers. The mixed response of managers to the causes and the need for intervention in interprofessional conflict, the awareness of its origins in shortage of resources, and a quiet confidence in the commitment of the staff to patient care, is perhaps best illuminated by the closing comments of one manager:

> *Unit general manager*: I think if there are tensions it probably relates to the pressure on both groups of staff. In my mind tension is healthy as long as it is controlled and as long as there is a mechanism for dealing with it if it gets out of hand. But I don't read any particular problems here that have a significant impact on what we are all trying to do, of delivering health care. There are too many committed people for that.

Clinical directorates

A new management unit, the clinical directorate, was being increasingly introduced during the course of our fieldwork, which sought to reintegrate some of these fragmented functions. The following discussion of clinical directorates, while initially based on evidence from our study, ranges into some considerations of possible further developments of this form of local governance.

Clinical directorates are management units which bring together a specialty, such as medicine, or a sub-specialty such as gynaecology and obstetrics (maternity). Each directorate has its own budget, and seeks contracts with purchasers to supply hospital services. Directorates have been in place in some British hospitals for several years, but the NHS reforms have encouraged their formation, so that directorates are an increasingly common feature of hospital organisation. Directorates were developed at the Johns Hopkins Hospital at Baltimore, USA, and arose from a recognition that, while hospital costs are largely determined as a result of decisions made by, or authorised by, senior doctors, doctors were only marginally involved in the management of hospital budgets. Structures vary in detail, but each directorate has a management structure that involves a clinical director, as yet, invariably a doctor, a nurse manager, and a business manager. The lines of accountability can be confusing; it is not unknown for a nurse manager of one directorate to double up as a business manager for another, or for a business manager to have unit management responsibilities as well. Since directorates were developed specifically in order to relate medical decision making to cost management, there is an issue as to the extent to which nursing will be able to hold on to a degree of professional autonomy when directorates, with medical directors, are the normal unit of clinical management.

Between 1966 and 1984 the nursing profession gained a greater level of autonomous control through the development of line management structures. At the start, this process was seen as the assertion of a distinct agenda for nursing in contrast to an era of strong medical influence. By 1984, when the Griffiths reform introduced the principle of general management, nursing was striving unsuccessfully to retain an autonomous line management structure separate to that of general managers. So nursing had no sooner cleared a space for itself relatively free from medical power, when general managers moved in to assert control over many aspects of nursing activity. Levitt and Wall (1992) suggest that the good times for nursing are over and gone, and the future, in the shape of general managers at the top, and medically dominated clinical directorates lower down, does not bode well for the nursing profession. A pessimistic view of nursing might observe that in the past 25 years the profession had a brief taste of power, while chief nursing officers were on the management teams, until the 1984 general management reforms demoted them. 'At a lower level in the organisation, the development of clinical directorates are seen by some nurses as a threat to their professional status because ward nurses are obliged to be much more accountable to the clinical directors, who are invariably doctors' (Levitt and Wall, 1992: 232). However, this may be an unduly gloomy prediction. An interesting feature of the directorate structure is that it is remarkably similar to the tri-partite grouping that dominated UK hospitals prior to the Griffiths reforms, forming the consensual management that Griffiths was credited with destroying. If nursing had its golden days in the era of consensual management, it is possible that the clinical directorates may bring a smaller, and maybe livelier, version of that kind of approach to hospital unit management, so that nursing might re-emerge from a painful decade with increased significance.

Nevertheless, our study found that some nurses were uneasy about certain aspects of clinical directorates, as were some consultants. A consultant's fears were the reverse of the nurse manager's.

> *Consultant*: Nursing staff think they will be eligible for directorships in the future, and I wouldn't take instruction from them!

> *Nurse manager*: I for one intend to compete in three years time against the consultants . . . and yes, I think this will cause quite a lot of ill feeling between nursing and medical staff.

We found other nurse managers who were optimistic that directorates would lead to better teamwork with medical colleagues, while most senior doctors showed little interest in the topic. Christine Hancock, RCN General Secretary, sees the essential issue as that of accountability:

> The key concept – inadequately understood – appears to be one of multiple accountability, where many people, especially professional practitioners, are accountable to different people for different things. Nurses are accountable to managers . . . to doctors, to their colleagues and to patients. Normally these accountabilities do not conflict . . . On the rare occasions when [they] conflict, primacy must be given to the interest of the patient or client. (Hancock, 1991: 3–5)

At a grassroots level, mundane and self-motivated issues were given rather more attention. What would happen to the existing nurse managers, and who would control ward-level appointments? Would consultants try to regain control of the nursing agenda by contriving to abolish the nurse manager grade, and insisting on having a final say over ward sister appointments? Nurse managers were well aware that consultants did not generally view them favourably. In the interviews we conducted with unit general managers there was evidence that consultants were indeed trying to influence the management structure so that nurse manager posts disappeared.

Unit general manager: A lot of doctors don't see the need for senior nurse managers 'Why are they there, they're not doing useful things on the ward, they're not helping me with my patients, and they are not helping centrally with management, so where do they fit in?' That's an attitude . . . that comes from a lot of different quarters . . .

Unit general manager: I need to define what [nurse managers] are doing, which I share with my senior nurse . . . She is extremely enthusiastic about her management role.

An equally contentious issue concerns appointments to ward sister grade posts. Given the bitterness of some of the comments made by consultants, and the accounts we were given by nurse managers, this is likely to be a significant area of contention. Consultants, acting through the clinical director, may well claim a right to influence, or even control, the appointment of ward sisters on the grounds that it is important that the ward sister conforms to the corporate values of the directorate. Nurses see this as an alibi for regaining medical control over a nursing agenda. It is the ward sister who supplies professional leadership and support to the nurses who give direct patient care. If the ward sister is inclined to support either a 'new nursing' or a 'medical model' of care, the ward is likely to move in the same direction. If consultants control ward nursing appointments, the trend is expected to be toward a strengthening of medical values. For many nurses, whether or not nursing retains control over nurse appointments is a litmus test of whether nursing will be able to preserve some professional autonomy.

Our conclusion is that nursing will at least maintain its position in the introduction of clinical directorates, not because of any unique claim to power, but because the nursing profession, unlike the medical profession, is well accustomed to a managerial ethos. The move to a clinical directorate structure will impose considerable strains on ward sisters, who will have to acquire new skills in managing a ward budget, but it does not require a paradigm shift of cultural values for the profession, but a downward delegation of responsibilities from the directorate nurse manager to the 'ward manager', that is, the ward sister recreated in a different role. If the directorate nurse managers are given adequate support from the director of nursing, and they in turn can offer effective support to ward sisters, then the experience of the profession within the directorates should be a positive one. The levels of support from the directorate nursing and business managers to ward staff will be crucial, as will the extent of funding pressure.

Heyssel et al. (1984) reports favourably from Baltimore. The clinical directorate system:

has attracted competent nurse managers who can advocate the role of nursing to administrators . . . They are capable of managing large numbers of people, budgeting resources appropriately, developing strong head nurse leaders, and evaluating the capability of nurses for promotion. The outcome has been joint decision making in the best interest of the entire functional unit. (Heyssel, 1984: 1477–80 as cited in Hancock, 1991: 3–5)

Medicine, by contrast, is having to move from a collegiate ethic, to a more corporate one, with a new emphasis on joint decision making and peer group assessment that does not fit easily with the individualism that has been characteristic of UK hospital consultants. Medical culture has not esteemed management; to be 'a management type' is to be inferior. Clinical directorates were designed to draw medicine into a central managerial role, but the medical profession over the past decade has frequently contested managerial power. There is a question as to whether the clinical directors become medical managers and then develop cultural values distinct from those of their clinical colleagues.

There is a debate within the United States as to whether medical managers are primarily concerned with the interests of their corporate sponsors or their professional colleagues. Elston (1991) supports the view developed by Friedson (1986):

Supervisory doctors . . . retain the values of and commitment to their profession, but at the same time, collegial relations are being altered. Thus the identification of some physicians as having entrepreneurial or managerial responsibility and not others, is, he suggests, driving a wedge into the principle of collegiality, of a community of autonomous peers at a local level. Institutionalised professional autonomy is being maintained through continued medical control over the supervision and management of medical care, even though some individual doctor's technical autonomy is being eroded. (Elston 1991: 74)

There is a central difference in the relative influence of medicine in the US and in the UK. Purchasing of the clinical services of consultant doctors working in hospitals is heavily influenced by general practitioner doctors, and public health consultants working in the community. The Elston and Friedson analysis, that the involvement of doctors in management represents a different form of medical control, rather than a loss of control to general managers, seems to be even more the case in the UK, where GPs have gained a more dominant position as the result of the NHS changes. Quite apart from any direct influence as a budget holder, GPs are involved in determining the purchasing decisions of health authorities. The medical profession therefore dominates both the purchasing and the providing aspects of health services, but ironically has less autonomy than before because the contracting system compels both GPs and consultants to conform to contractual arrangements, unless there is sufficient money in the health authority budget to pay for extra-contractual referrals. Toward the end of a financial year this is often not the case. The significant cultural change in hospital medicine is therefore likely to be the loss of collegiality, and the growth of medical managerialism.

Even so, this is a significant cultural change. There was limited evidence in the many discussions we conducted with consultants that it will happen lightly. It is difficult to believe that the most ambitious consultants will be eager to become clinical directors, but if these posts are filled by consultants seen as less prestigious, how will they adjudicate the rival claims of eminent colleagues? Will the clinical directors find themselves in the kind of position described to us by ward and theatre sisters, of being caught in the crossfire between competing consultants? If so, and it seems probable, then the clinical director may find a unity of purpose with senior nursing colleagues and business managers, taking part in consensual management and having to accommodate and control the power of individual consultants. As yet there is little evidence as to how clinical directorates are developing, though there are some suggestions that consultant reluctance to share decision making is reducing the impact of the directorates.

One aspect of patient care and ward management that is being influenced by the development of directorates is the issue of admitting patients to wards that belong to a different specialty, when some wards are full, i.e. 'outlier' or 'boarded out' patients. With each specialty having its own budget, and seeking its own income, there is a greater reluctance to send patients to other specialties, or to receive 'outliers' that block directorate beds. This may have an impact on admissions, but it is likely to improve care for those admitted.

The array of directorates within a hospital corresponds to the nature of the service contracts agreed between the district health authorities, and GP budget holders as purchasers of health care services, and the hospitals which provide those services. Medical wards in a typical district general hospital admit a large proportion of their patients as emergencies, and many are elderly. Contracts for medical and elderly care services are commonly issued as block contracts, and the likelihood is that in smaller hospitals medicine and elderly care will be grouped together to form one directorate, though in specialist and teaching hospitals other structural patterns may emerge. Surgical contracts, by contrast, are commonly 'cost and volume' contracts for specialties that admit many of their patients from waiting lists, and may become more precisely costed, based on a cost per case formula. The impact of contracts will be significantly different for a medical directorate with a reasonably secure locally based block contract, compared to a surgical specialty having to compete for waiting list referrals, with correspondingly different cultural values emerging for each kind of directorate. How interprofessional team working will emerge within the different specialties remains to be seen.

'Consumers'

While management has traditionally been focused on the relations between workers and their bosses, new wave management theory has insisted on the greater importance of the relationship of workers and their customers. Within this theory, this relationship has typically been seen as most effectively mediated via the market. However, there are other ways in which consumers can make their preferences known, through users' groups, pressure groups, statutory organisations to represent patients, and through democratic structures.

Examples of consumer pressure groups in health include: various groups to improve women's choice and control over their treatment during childbirth, such as the National Childbirth Trust and the Association for Improvements in Maternity Services; the National Association for the Welfare of Children in Hospital (NAWCH), founded in 1961 to improve the emotional welfare of children in hospital largely by demanding the acceptability of the presence of parents; and The Patients Association, founded in 1963, to oppose research on patients without their consent or knowledge (Williamson, 1992).

Community Health Councils (CHCs) have a statutory responsibility to represent all health service users in their district, providing an advice and information service, assistance to people who want to make complaints, and monitoring of health services provided. There is typically a staff of two who are assisted by around 24 volunteers, and who seek to represent the views of the residents of the health authority district. Watkins (1987) noted that the secretary (chief officer) of a CHC sets the tone for the work of local services. In the division that now exists between purchaser and provider, the CHC's role is similar to that of the health authority quality monitoring staff, but the involvement of lay members gives a grassroots perspective that is missing elsewhere in the NHS. Until the recent reforms, they had a statutory right to be consulted on ward closures and any significant change in service provision. In practice, their effectiveness varied considerably from district to district. Neuberger (1993) sees a similar variation in the new NHS structure.

The basic weakness of the patient's position as a consumer or customer is his or her lack of effective power. The GP and the district health authority have to act as a proxy for the patient in purchasing health care and, as part of this function, both are paying rather more attention to patients' preferences. This is welcome, but is far from satisfactory. The purchaser has no obligation to act on the information given by patients, and is unlikely to do so if this conflicts with institutional goals unless pressure for change is well argued, commands significant local support, and funding can be identified from elsewhere in the budget. Bartlett and LeGrand (1994: 66) see the democratic chain of accountability over Trusts as being 'both long and weak'.

The increased attention given to the outcomes of treatment may in practice give greater benefits to patients but, characteristically, organised patient involvement in developing user indicators of successful outcomes is almost wholly undeveloped (Neuberger, 1993).

Within hospitals, there is a question as to who best represents the patient on the ward. This issue arises particularly around the treatment and care of the terminally ill, discussed in Chapter 2. While doctors and nurses often take a joint and harmonious decision after consulting relatives, on some occasions there were divisions of opinion, with nurses considering that they were closer to the patient and more sensitive to his or her needs, while doctors considered that they were looking after the real needs of the patient as well. The development of primary nursing has given a boost to the claim by nurses that they are the patient's advocate.

The customers of doctors are seldom involved in medical audit. Joule (1992: 1) comments: 'Users have little access to the first stage of decision making on the selection of topics for audit. Complaints about clinical care are occasionally, though rarely, fed into the audit process. Throughout the next stages of the audit cycle which deal with setting criteria and standards, user involvement is similarly underdeveloped.'

Conclusion

Medicine, as a traditionally organised profession, has a mode of governance which has similarities with that advocated by new wave management. Nursing does not have the autonomy that is associated with the traditional form of a profession, and has had a form of governance more consistent with Taylorism, though recent changes demonstrate a movement away from this. These different modes of governance coexist in adjacent occupations in the same workplace. Though there are striking parallels between the theories of the management of employment and the nature of the organisation of health professionals, it is not complete. The main exception is that of the organisation of the highly skilled, yet quite regimented, work of nursing. The conclusion must be that highly skilled work does not necessarily take the autonomous form presumed by many theorists.

The emphasis that is increasingly given to the management of professional skill-mix demonstrates the existence of an invigorated form of Taylorism located at the level of hospital personnel management, but the speed of change, and the implementation of change by individual Trusts is sufficiently variable to impel caution in pronouncing on the nature of NHS employment within hospitals. While there has been devolution of some authority to Trusts, as yet there is little firm evidence that there is a genuine devolution of authority to the directorates or ward level staff, though responsibility for budgetary control has been devolved. Hence our belief that the present pattern is most aptly described as devolved Taylorism.

The devolution of the management of health professionals down to the level of the ward or directorate, when it occurs, necessitates a reconsideration of the issues involved in the organisation of professions. Such devolution requires professionals to negotiate with each other the solution to practical problems for patients rather than referring these decisions up their professional hierarchies. The ward or directorate team is necessarily interprofessional. Thus the devolution inherent in the new wave forms of management necessitates close interprofessional working.

Studies of single professions are out of date if the new forms of working practice are to be understood, though an understanding of, and a respect for, the cultural differences of individual professions is essential. The complexity of the coexistence of differing lines of accountability are inherent in modern hospitals. The new team unit is the ward or directorate, not the profession, if the outcome of the best patient care is to be given priority.

6

Post-Fordism and the Health Professions

We began this book with questions about the changing nature of employment that we sought to answer by looking at the work of doctors and nurses since highly skilled workers, such as professionals, were expected by many social theorists to be the workers of the future. Why are teams of such professional staff seen to be in such urgent need of being 'managed'? Is this new wave management, with its stress on devolving responsibility to semi-autonomous institutions, an appropriate approach to public services dominated by professionals? Are professions self-interested organisations, lacking a proper focus on their customers? Do the new forms of organisation warrant the use of the term 'post-Fordist'? The interprofessional relations of medicine and nursing seen as a key test ground for these issues.

In investigating these interprofessional relations, we found that the boundaries between the responsibilities of medical and nursing staff were, not unexpectedly, the source of some tensions. We expected these boundaries to show evidence of the strains of competitive occupations in constant adjustment due to changing technology and the position of such groups in the wider society, as well as their corporate occupational strategies for collective advancement. Indeed, we saw the attempt by nurses to resist subordination to medicine and to develop new skills as part of a professionalisation strategy. There were times when each profession engaged in demarcation disputes and the interests of patients did not always determine the outcome of conflicts, though there were more examples of interprofessional collaboration. However, there was no simple process of doctors resisting nurses' strategy of professional advancement; doctors were as often pleased if nurses developed technical skills which enhanced the work on which doctors needed to draw, though they were more resistant if the changes involved nurses' control over the organisation of the ward. In a curiously symmetrical manner some nurses were reluctant to take on new responsibilities for fear that it would merely add to their workload or that it would lead to greater divisions within the nursing profession. The ambiguity and variability in whether there was competition or cooperation between doctors and nurses makes theories of professional organisation predominantly in terms of direct self-interest too simple. Doctors have an interest in the competence of 'their' nurses, since they depend on them to carry out their shared goal of healing the patient. The ostensible boundary of the nurse 'caring' and the doctor 'treating' was in practice a fuzzy and negotiable one played by each group according to the circumstances. These boundaries were generally well negotiated by the staff caring directly for patients on most occasions. Devolving authority to ward-based teams in new wave management style appeared to be an entirely feasible option, and one that would benefit the delivery of care.

When the pressures on staff were examined a different aspect of professional work emerged. The focus on the output of the hospital in terms of numbers treated was leading to a fragmentation of the ward-based team. Extra patients to raise bed occupancy rates were fitted in in ways which broke up the cohesive ward-based teams and raised frictions over admissions and discharge procedures. There was a contradiction between the desire for higher throughput typical of Taylorist management and a Fordist regime, and the patient-centred, ward-based, cohesive interprofessional team more appropriate to new wave management and post-Fordism. If the patient, as consumer, is the centre with individuated packages of care, then Taylorist management is inappropriate. The tension between these coexisting logics of organisation was evident in many issues in the hospital.

Conflicts between Fordist and post-Fordist principles underlay many of the tensions between hospital workers. This is the best way to understand the changing relations of employment, the changing relations between consumers and producers, and the forms of state regulation of such social relations in contemporary Britain, and many other Western countries. We see, however, not a simple transition from one logic to another, but rather their uneasy coexistence.

There is more than one theory of post-Fordism. In the golden post-Fordist scenario it is considered that everyone benefits from its development: consumers have products more closely tailored to their needs; workers have greater autonomy and both enjoy their work and work better; resources are used more efficiently; employers make more profits. The key feature is the belief that human resources are central to production and that if work is organised so as to enable workers to use the full range of their human attributes everyone will benefit (Piore and Sabel, 1984). However, in the more pessimistic versions of the thesis, there is a prediction merely of new forms of exploitation of workers under new forms of capitalist relations (Aglietta, 1987). In the versions of the thesis which contain a compromise between the two, we have the golden scenario for core workers and for consumers, but a pessimistic scenario of increased casualisation of employment for those on the periphery (Atkinson, 1986; Handy, 1990).

The debates on post-Fordism are diverse and the distinctions between the various versions of the post-Fordist thesis are important in assessing whether it is consistent with the changes in health work. The element common to them all is that there is a transformation of employment relations so as to create a layer of job-enriched functionally flexible workers. The key point of divergence is whether all workers are to be up-skilled during the change, or whether there is a simultaneous creation of a less skilled periphery with insecure contracts of employment. Atkinson's model has a periphery of numerically flexible less skilled workers, absent in the more optimistic scenario of Piore and Sabel. These workers bear the brunt of the fluctuating demand for labour and are employed on less secure contracts, sometimes part-time, sometimes sub-contracted from the main employer. Atkinson's model of flexibility is thus one in which only some workers, those in the core, benefit from upskilling and a more diverse range of tasks, unlike Piore and Sable who posit more universal benefits.

This significant divergence of view between writers on ostensibly the same topic stems from profound differences in their underlying theory of social relations. Aglietta (1987) considers that social relations are inherently antagonistic when there is one group owning property, while Piore and Sabel (1984) do not consider the ownership of property to be quite such a significant determinant of social relations. While all these post-Fordist theorists see the relations between producers and consumers as more important than many earlier writers, it is Piore and Sabel who see the consumer desire for varied goods and services as most causally significant; for Aglietta the problem is the inability of consumers to consume the goods produced; while consumers are less prominent in the work of Atkinson.

One of the contested points in the debate over the post-Fordist thesis has been over whether there is empirical evidence of changes in employment relations which substantiates the thesis. Pollert and her collaborators in the Warwick School have vigorously denied that the changes which are occurring constitute sufficiently new phenomena to justify these claims (Pollert, 1991), taking particular issue with the version of the flexibility thesis represented in the work of Atkinson (1986). Pollert argues that the changes are primarily those in the interpretation of industrial relations and stem from the revival of neo-classical economics and its focus on flexibility and that there is insufficient evidence to justify claims that there is a new polarisation into a core and a peripheral workforce, arguing instead that these are merely a continuing feature of capitalism. Pollert's position is echoed by most of the contributors in her book, for instance, Marginson (1991), using data from large private manufacturers from 1985, suggests that the extent of temporary and indirect forms of employment has not significantly changed, and Elger (1991), using data on manufacturing, suggests that job enlargement and work intensification, rather than the more benign phenomenon of functional flexibility has occurred. However, there are some who disagree (Whittington, 1991). Other evidence suggests that there has been a considerable increase in flexible work practices, including Hakim's (1987a) analyses of UK statistics, Standing's (1989) claims that flexibility has become a global phenomenon among industrialised countries and various case studies (Jessop et al., 1991 and Lash and Urry, 1987).

The post-war NHS

Several aspects of the immediate post-war history of health work have been driven by a Fordist logic, partly as a consequence of state intervention. This is seen in attempts to centralise, the development of less skilled specialist occupations, and the creation of a simpler, clearer hierarchy of command. Three important examples of this are: first, the creation of the National Health Service itself in 1946; secondly, the development of specialist health occupations with a very narrow range of tasks in the period following the Second World War; thirdly, the introduction of general management following the Griffiths Report in 1983.

The first, and most obvious, instance of Fordism was the act of nationalisation itself in 1946, a political decision imposing a single central national authority, with a hierarchy ultimately rising to the Health Minister. Its key, and proudest, feature was universal provision with no distinction between patients. There was a drive to create a uniform level of service between previously disparate regions. It involved the negotiation of national terms of service for health workers (see Klein, 1989; Stacey, 1988).

Secondly, there were many detailed ways in which the Fordist logic worked, for instance, in the creation of ever more specialised sub-occupations, with specific training. The movement of task boundaries is a continuous process. Historically change has been led by the medical profession, though this is changing so that managers are currently the more active players in initiating change. When the medical profession considered that a task had become routine they then sought to transfer it (dump it – some would say) to the nursing staff. If the nursing profession successfully resisted this transference, for whatever reason, or if the task was seen to be too technical to be the responsibility of nurses, a specialist group emerged, responsible for a very narrow range of specific tasks. An example of a task absorbed by nursing is the recording of blood pressures, once the prerogative of doctors, and now done routinely by junior nurses in training or, we have observed, by newly appointed health support workers. We have described the pressure on nurses to take over the administration of intravenous drugs in a similar way.

More Fordist logic is seen in the taking of blood samples. These samples are taken for analysis to provide indications of levels and nature of infection, blood cell counts, blood plasma analysis, and levels of vitamins, hormones and other constituents. Taking blood has traditionally been a junior doctor's job. However, for some time now hospital authorities have handed over this task to people who they train specifically and solely to take blood samples, a group called phlebotomists. In most hospitals nurses are not allowed to take bloods, though the majority of staff are fully aware that nurses are far more qualified than the phlebotomists who are coming round the wards taking bloods. The technical task is simple, and dangerous complications are much less likely than in the case of IVs despite the apparent similarity of the technical side of the procedure. This is a task which is considered too simple for nurses to want to take on as a duty, yet one which reverts to the junior doctor rather than to the nurse if the specialist phlebotomist is unavailable. The logic of this might not appear entirely clear. Even so, it is not the only instance of a task which falls between the junior doctor and the trained nurse in this way. The issue of taking bloods can be better understood in the context of the large number of small specialist occupations which have developed in hospitals for tasks which are considered, for one reason or another, to fall outside the boundaries of either doctors or nurses. There are further examples of this.

Cardiology technicians and operating department assistants are used to provide technical support to doctors in areas where the work is considered to be both too routine and too technical to be either a medical or a nursing task. The operating department assistants developed because the work was not suitable for either a staff nurse or an enrolled nurse, and because it was technical (hence inappropriate for a largely female workforce?), related not to patients, but to machines. Operating department assistants are paid on a technical grade, together with phlebotomists and path lab technicians. There are many small occupations such as these, each with its own bargaining system. The history of hospital medicine is replete with the proliferation of small specialist occupations (see, for instance, Witz, 1992).

Thirdly, the introduction of general managers after the 1983 Griffiths Report is perhaps one of the highest profile introductions of Fordist techniques into the NHS, again as a result of a political decision (Butler, 1992; Flynn, 1992; Owens and Glennerster, 1990; Strong and Robinson, 1990). This was discussed in some detail in Chapter 5, showing the varying effects that this has had on the organisation of medicine and nursing.

The 1980s and 1990s

A general move towards Fordist practices characterised the post-war period in health until the early 1980s, and has since been replaced by an attempt to shift health work in a post-Fordist direction. However, there are several major qualifications: first, there is a considerable difference in the extent to which different occupations have been affected by these changes; secondly, the implementation of the post-Fordist drive has met some serious barriers relating to the problems of markets in the NHS; thirdly these moves have not replaced Taylorist style management. The two uneasily coexist, with individual Trust variations.

Many of these developments are politically led, with the initiative coming from the national government. This lends support to the notion of post-Fordism being a more societal phenomenon, but not to the versions of the thesis driven more by economics. The extent to which finance is a motor for change is controversial. It is repeatedly claimed by government that this is the case, but since the NHS is one of the cheapest systems of health care in Western countries, this is a problematic claim (Butler, 1992; Ham, 1992; Harrison et al., 1990).

An ostensible drive to decentralisation may be perceived in the creation of the opted-out Trusts. The Trusts should be more flexible because of their greater autonomy from the national system, and their ability to respond more directly to consumer needs. The new system of internal competition was intended to make these reformed organisations more orientated to the needs of patients. However, the extent of this autonomy and participation in free markets is still unresolved. Further, the reduction in hospital beds in London following the Tomlinson Report is to take place on the basis of planning and politics, as much as on markets (Butler, 1992; Ham, 1992; Harrison et al., 1990). Since then the market has succeeded in destabilising the hospitals that were recommended for retention by Tomlinson. The London picture thus shows two incompatible systems limiting the ability of either to function consistently. As we saw in Chapter 4, these processes are limited by the pressure to keep up the throughput of patient numbers and the budgetary disciplines generated by the market.

Markets in health

Markets are not simply natural phenomena; they require regulation in order to make them work. This regulation has long been a concern of US economists (see Majone, 1990). There are long-established discussions of the ways to deal with the provision of the information necessary to make markets work, and over the nature and number of regulatory bodies to reduce fraud and associated market failures (Kay and Vickers, 1990). US health economists make clear that competition does not necessarily lead to greater efficiency (Light, 1990a,b).

Recent management theory and practice has tried to combine the pressure and efficiency of the market by bringing market pressures down to as many levels of the organisation as possible, while bestowing levels of autonomy which make people feel in control and thus more prepared to work hard. This has involved tight financial regulation, but more autonomy for individual workers as to how they achieve these financial targets. This is being introduced into not only the private sector, but the public sector too. One of the apparent paradoxes of the recent changes to the NHS is that of local–central relations. On the one hand, there is devolution of funding down to hospitals and GPs; on the other, there is strong central control of the level of funding and of this mode of managerial control. The same has occurred in education with the devolution of budgets to schools (Deem and Brehony, 1993). The trend to the devolution of budgets generates conflicts, particularly when it is in the context of tight budgets. Devolution by itself would not necessarily generate such conflict; it is the context of restraint that leads to strife.

This issue is highly relevant to the new wave management interest in the 'tight and loose' strategy. New wave management literature has emphasised the efficiency of the 'tight and loose'. This rather contradictory phrase captures the notion of central control over budget allocation with decentralised decision making over its spending. It is considered to give more autonomy to lower level workers, and hence more scope for their innovation, than the older more bureaucratic forms of management.

The irony of the new managerialism, or new wave management, in the NHS, is that while it captures some progressive impulses in its orientation to consumers and clients, decentralisation of decision making, and less hierarchical organisation; simultaneously, it has regressive leanings in a tendency to undermine a public service ethic and a focus on financial limits. Other tendencies are either inherently contradictory or neutral such as: encouraging innovation; stimulating entrepreneurial action within an organisation; breaking with tradition. The creation of markets has similar contradictory aspects in that, on the one hand, it encourages a monetarisation of worth; while, on the other, it can support a focus on the consumer or client; other aspects are contradictory or neutral, for example, widening access, albeit only to those who have the appropriate currency.

Some forms of post-Fordism are considered to increase workers' autonomy. This is clearly not happening to all workers in NHS hospitals. At one level of analysis the introduction of managers and markets appears to follow the same trajectory. In fact, they lead in contradictory directions in the NHS.

Public sector markets are not real markets because there is no potential for real growth. They cannot bring in more business. They have too much business already, queues of eager customers on waiting lists. Furthermore, a provider unit that is successful in attracting more 'customers', that is, patients, will have to be told to stop doing so, if, as often happens, a department succeeds and treats more patients than it is required to treat under the terms of its contracts. Attracting more customers is very different from attracting more contracts. The promise that was held out to staff when the market system was introduced, namely that 'money would follow the patient', has turned out largely to mean that patients cannot move unless money precedes patients.

In the evaluation of the introduction of quasi-markets in social policy more generally, LeGrand and Bartlett (1993) suggest that there are four criteria by which the success of this innovation should be assessed. These are the increase of efficiency, responsiveness, choice and equity. These are considered more likely to be achieved if the market structure facilitates competition, if there is sufficient information to enable the market to run effectively, that the costs of the complex transaction are not too high, that motivation is present, and that 'cream-skimming' or adverse selection is avoided. Their conclusion is that these are variably present in the different areas of social policy and with different aspects of the quasi-markets in health.

Bourne and Ezzamel (1986, 1987) have addressed some of these concerns about the specificity of health work in relation to the theories of new wave managers. They also use these theories to understand new management regimes in relation to health workers, setting out some modifications they think necessary. Bourne and Ezzamel have argued that Peters and Waterman (1982) are insufficiently aware of the specific contexts of decision making. They argue that a more sophisticated approach is needed to transaction costs than the simple assumption made by Peters and Waterman that the market is the most efficient way of allocating resources. The transaction cost approach (Jones, 1983; Ouchi, 1980,1981; Wilkins and Ouchi, 1983) examines the costs and relative efficiency of three mechanisms of corporate organisation: markets, hierarchies (or bureaucracies) and corporate cultures (or clans) (Bourne and Ezzamel, 1986: 205). These different modes of organisation have different efficiencies according to whether the context in which they exist has the following two criteria: first, an unambiguous way of measuring individual performance, secondly, a congruence between the goals of employer and employee. Bourne and Ezzamel's three mechanisms of corporate organisation relate to the criteria of performance ambiguity and goal incongruence as shown in Table 6.1.

Table 6.1   *Transaction costs and corporate governance*

	Organisational characteristics		
Ambiguity of individual performance measurement	Low	Moderately high	Very high
Extent of goal incongruence between employer and employee	Variable	Moderately high	Low
	Most efficient exchange mechanism is a market	Most efficient exchange is mediated through a hierarchy	Most efficient exchange is organised through clan culture

Source: Bourne and Ezzamel, 1986

Bourne and Ezzamel criticise Peters and Waterman on the grounds that their argument is not sensitive to context. Markets are supposed to be efficient if there is low ambiguity of performance indicators, despite high levels of goal incongruence. If performance ambiguity and goal incongruence are moderately high, then markets are seen as inefficient because of the effort needed to monitor and control. In these circumstances, hierarchies are more efficient because they rely on employment contracts which are incompletely written. When ambiguity of performance evaluation is very high, but goal incongruence is low, the most efficient is that of clan or corporate culture. This is because markets fail under the need for tight specification of contracts and performance which is unforthcoming. Likewise hierarchies fail because of the difficulties of monitoring performance. Instead the culture bonds people together in trust relations.

Bourne and Ezzamel applied this analysis to the NHS before the introduction of markets, though their arguments remain relevant. They argue that the NHS is characterised by a low degree of goal incongruence, that is, most people broadly agree on its objectives. In contrast, performance measurement is very difficult and that instruments for this are undeveloped (1986: 120). Further, they argue that the Griffiths initiative was problematic because it did not sufficiently distinguish the context and management needs of the public sector (in this case, the NHS) from that of the private sector, such as Sainsbury's (see also Flynn, 1990; Light, 1990a,b). The NHS has traditionally operated on the basis of a corporate culture in which clinical freedom is a central value. This clinical freedom has nevertheless been subject to a number of constraints, such as legal, ethical and religious controls. There have been attempts, such as the 1979 Royal Commission, the Cogwheel reports (see DHSS, 1972), case mix analysis, and the resource management initiative, to involve doctors in financial accountability. However, these attempts have sometimes led to a polarisation of views within the medical profession between clinical freedom which is associated with caring, and financial accountability which is seen negatively as of inferior importance and counter to the interests of the patient.

Bourne and Ezzamel conclude that, in the absence of reliable measures of individual performance, the introduction of the Griffiths recommendations was likely to lead to more ritualistic than rationalistic modes of control. That is, the type of management Griffiths recommended depends on a support network of financial information which does not exist. Hence the general management system introduced by Griffiths could not be a form of rational control. Rather, we have merely another clan, with its own views. Bourne and Ezzamel introduce some much needed specificity into the models of organisations put forward by Peters and his colleagues. In contrast, Bourne and Ezzamel (1987) argue in favour of devolved budgeting as the process most likely to reduce the high levels of performance ambiguity. It is seen as a potentially success-ful compromise between management and professional autonomy, and they implicitly reject the view that this is a necessary contradic-tion. They suggest that academic and clinical freedom can be maintained while attention is paid to financial issues.

The criticism that Bourne and Ezzamel use against Peters and Waterman can be applied also to their analysis; it is insufficiently context specific. In treating the NHS as a whole entity, they have understated the contrasts that exist between different organisational units of the health service, so that they do not address the possibility that markets may be efficient NHS mechanisms in some contexts, and inefficient in others.

In the internal health market, contracts between health authori-ties and provider units are normally one of three types: block contracts, cost and volume contracts, and cost per case contracts. The last of these is the form of contract that fits most closely to a market model, while block contracts resemble a more bureaucratic arrangement. The Department of Health has encouraged health authorities to move away from block contracts, and towards cost per case contracts (Neumann, et al., 1990). If Bourne and Ezzamel's analysis of the relationship between performance ambiguity, goal incongruence and the effectiveness of markets holds true, then there should be some pattern in the use of the different kinds of contracts and different areas of hospital activity.

Emergency health care generates a high level of goal congruence; put more simply, staff 'pull together' when they are providing an emergency service. The staff in the surgical unit at Central hospital, discussed in Chapter 4, make just that point. A market in emerg-ency care is unnecessary as a way of motivating staff. Performance ambiguity may be high, in that it is difficult to monitor individual performance, and impossible to predict demand on performance accurately. Leaving aside for the moment any discussion of the ethics of a market in emergency hospital care, the transaction costs of such an enterprise are such that a bureaucratic or clan culture form of organisation are more appropriate. Using Bourne and Ezzamel's analysis it would be reasonable to expect that emergency hospital care would not fit a market model. This is acknowledged within the internal market structure, in that emergency referrals by GPs are outside the budget holding financial system, and hospital emergency services are covered by a block contract from health authorities, rather than a cost per case or a cost and volume contract.

Waiting list surgery (i.e. 'cold' surgery) is different in so far as transaction costs are considered. Markets exist for specific operations, both by encouraging competition between hospitals, and by using the facilities of private hospitals. Patients can travel for 'cold' surgery in a way that is impossible for emergency care. The market compels attention on to costs, output and the quality of services, rather than the inclinations of providers. Recovery rates and items of cost can be very precisely compared, so that performance ambiguity may be low. There may be high goal incongruence in the sense that different values are given to the relative merits of innovative and routine operations, of some specialties compared to others, and of purchasing many low cost or fewer high cost operations. Consultant employees may wish to develop or retain operative procedures for which an epidemiological justification is weak, or want to develop skills for which there is a demand in the private sector. The pattern of low performance ambiguity, and varying levels of goal congruence fits in to Bourne and Ezzamel's description of an activity that can be effectively managed through a market mechanism, and this is reflected in the pricing system used for surgical contracts. Within the NHS contracts for surgery are either cost and volume or cost per case. Private hospitals use cost per case pricing, and this has provided a model for NHS pricing.

A consideration of transaction costs alone would therefore suggest that waiting list surgery could be incorporated into a market mechanism, but that emergency care may be more efficiently provided within a pattern of organisation controlled through a clan culture. The seemingly obvious flaw in this statement is that NHS hospitals exist to provide both emergency and 'cold' surgery, so the advantage of a market in 'cold' surgery has to be balanced by the inappropriateness of a market mechanism in a service that has a large element of emergency provision. In effect, two systems are running concurrently, an internal market for waiting list surgery, and a more bureaucratic system for financing emergency hospital systems. Tensions between them are a noticeable feature of the NHS; transferring an orthopaedic contract for waiting list surgery has an immediate effect on the viability of trauma and orthopaedic departments, and this in turn has an impact on the stability of the accident and emergency department.

Resources for the provision of health care in the NHS have long fallen short of demand for these services. Historically, this shortfall has been dealt with by rationing and waiting lists. The new system locates the problem of the shortfall differently. The market is supposed to allocate resources more efficiently between provider units, but cannot deal with the absolute shortfall, except by a marginal reduction in costs. 'Market' pressures would lead to the closure of the more expensive hospitals.

The debates on markets in health now involve complex considerations as to which units should be constructed as players, and which
issues of resource allocation should be placed through markets and
which by administrative decision. Many countries now run systems
in which there are markets at certain places, but not at others, with
sophisticated regulation of their working (see Saltman and von
Otter, 1992). Most policy debates are no longer about either
planning or markets, but rather how several versions of each are to
be integrated into a complex whole. A pattern whereby purchasers
and providers are linked by long-term, non-competitive contracts
might make more possible a stable and equitable distribution of
health care facilities. Such an arrangement could facilitate devolution to smaller units without the instability and fragmentation
generated by competitive markets.

Different groups of workers have been variously affected by these
developments. Indeed, when the view is widened beyond the
doctors and nurses which have so far been the focus of this book,
this is even more strongly the case. Managerialisation has variously
reorganised different groups of workers. Ancillary workers have
been subject to a process of peripheralisation best described in the
theories of Atkinson (1986) and Handy (1990), in that they have
been separated from the main employer by a process of sub-
contracting. This is quite different from the treatment of both
doctors and nurses.

A quite different interpretation of the decision not to make
patients the purchasers within the market, is that, if health care
is simultaneously to remain free at the point of delivery, and if, as is
believed, the demand for health care greatly exceeds supply, it is
necessary to control spending. The US literature on cost containment in health care is instructive (see Davis et al., 1990).

The 'consumer'

What does the 'consumer' mean in health? This is a concept which
derives its meaning from contexts which are entirely unlike the
public sector health service. Much of the more optimistic post-
Fordist literature has suggested that there can be a progressive
dimension to the elevation of the consumer. This includes the
possibility of consumer choice and the creation of diversity, as seen
especially in the work of Piore and Sabel (1984), and the work of the
'new times' theorists (Hall and Jacques, 1989). The possibility of
more carefully individualised packages of care to the benefit of
clients is stressed in the work of public sector management consultants (O'Higgins, 1992).

In the case of the introduction of markets or quasi-markets in health the issue is highly complex because of the lack of obvious and agreed referent to the content of 'market' and 'consumer'. The more populist applications of the terms are refused by the government. Popularly it might be presumed that the consumer is the patient. However, the markets that the government has set up turn the health authorities and the GP fund holders into the 'consumer' as purchaser, separated from provider units such as hospitals. That is, we see a split between the receiver of the services, the patient, and the purchaser of the services, the health authority and GP fund holder. This split between purchaser and recipient of services is unusual in relation to the normal use of the concept of 'consumer'.

There are a number of contenders for the title of consumer within health care in addition to the patient undergoing treatment. There are potential patients, such as sick people not undergoing treatment. These are people on lists waiting to enter hospital, as well as those with undiagnosed conditions which impair their health. There is the general public, which is the focus of the public health discourse and needs to be kept healthy through health education, healthy lifestyles and immunisation. As well as people who might be the targets of health intervention, there are the entities which have been constructed within the new internal market as customers. These are the district health authorities and GP fund holders which, as the purchasers of health care, are the customers of the provider units, such as hospitals.

These distinctions are not merely academic, but relate to real divisions of interest. For instance, we saw that the division between sick people on the ward and sick people not yet on the ward underlay the issue of admissions which could be a source of tension between hard-pressed nursing staff concerned with the patients already on their ward, and doctors who wished to admit sick people they had seen in outpatient clinics. Once a person has achieved the status of patient undergoing treatment there are various professional codes of conduct which prioritise their needs, embodied, for instance, in the Hippocratic oath of doctors. Not-yet-admitted sick people do not have advocates who are as powerfully present as those already on the ward.

The argument for not making the patient the purchaser within the new health market was that the patient could not have the knowledge to make appropriate choices. Indeed, they could have had vouchers, as was argued more generally for state services by the Public Choice political grouping on the Right. However, this would have taken power away from the centre as well as being difficult to operate in a context of variable risk. Again we see a key, but sometimes understated, aspect of markets being important. Markets need knowledge to make them function, in order that consumers/purchasers can make informed decisions. But how is the sick person, or potentially sick person, or simply a member of the public, to be represented as a consumer within the health care system if they are not competent to do this themselves? The solution produced by the government in the recent changes has been to have entities representing the consumer in health: the district health authorities and the GP fund holders. The impact of these changes is widely debated (Butler, 1992; Harrison et al., 1992; LeGrand and Bartlett, 1993).

However, there are other mechanisms by which consumers' interests can be represented. First, there are consumer movements within health, which have advocated particular changes in health policy. Secondly, there are Community Health Councils, which are bodies of local representatives who represent consumers. Thirdly, there is the issue of whether the patient's doctor or the patient's nurse can act effectively as the patient's advocate.

Consumerism has been a growing phenomenon in Britain and the West over the past 40 years and has a particular configuration within the NHS, where it includes a high value on patient autonomy relating to respect, support, information, control, choice and decision making. The health consumer movement is located at the confluence of three strands: the creation of a climate of scepticism; the popularising of disturbing accounts of professionals and institutions; the intense concern of particular groups of patients and patients' relatives (Williamson, 1992).

The balancing of the interests of patients who are already in hospital, and sick people who are not, is difficult. The shift of power within medicine from hospitals towards the community is a long run and very important change in health care. An important effect of the changes in the NHS has been to place control of choice between health care funding and health promotion outside the hospital.

Accountability

Accountability has been an ever present issue within the NHS, resolved in quite different ways in different periods. This has been associated with quite different relations between doctors, the state and patients. Before 1948 the medical profession had autonomy, but were constrained by patients' incomes. Before the NHS was established, doctors were accountable to themselves, working within a professional code of ethics, but compelled to limit the treatment that they ordered for particular patients to what was affordable, either through insurance or private income. In the period 1948–74, medicine became formally accountable to the state, but with a strong local element. Doctors were part of the controlling power, brought into the hospital boards as 'experts'. GPs remained independent contractors. Hospital doctors and nurses were accountable to the state, but not managed by the state.

Between 1974 and 1985 both medicine and nursing were accountable to a centralised state service, but in practice they largely controlled state medicine through their representation on management teams, and area and regional boards. The process of trying to involve doctors in budgetary control began as health care costs escalated. The pattern remained of formal accountability to central government, through the area and regional health authorities, but the professions dominated the management teams at each organisational level. There was something of a syndicalist structure, with the professions accountable to central government, but in practice controlling many aspects of service organisation. The professions began to monitor their performance, as for instance with the perioperative mortality survey, but retained control of such information. However, little attention was given to issues of professional management and evaluation of the outcomes of professional care. The existence of a form of professional syndicalism did not mean responsiveness to a notion of public accountability.

In the period 1985–91 medicine was both accountable to the state and managed by the state. There was an abrupt change with the introduction of general management principles, and greater use of budgetary control mechanisms, such as performance review, performance related pay, resource management initiatives, health authority reviews. The professions' ability to control the organisation of hospital and community services through their dominant position on management teams disappeared. The introduction of a nurse grading system in spite of professional resistance demonstrated the strength of a Taylorist management structure. GPs remained independent contractors, but state intrusion into their management began with limits on the lists of drugs that GPs could prescribe, indicative drugs budgets, payment targets for immunisation and some screening services.

Since 1991 professions have become accountable to semi-autonomous institutions through a managed market. The mechanisms for budgetary control are no longer imposed by central government because the need to win and maintain contracts has devolved these disciplines down to the Trusts, or health authority managed hospitals. There is still a central control structure, and the two forms of governance – markets and central planning – collide at times, notably in London. The introduction of a market has been accompanied by a greater emphasis on evaluating the outcomes of treatment, through systems of audit, though these are largely controlled by the professions. While some writers, notably Flynn (1992), have seen medical audit as part of a process of state managerialism, an alternative view is that audit could make professional work accountable to public scrutiny.

Loyalty is encouraged to the institution, not to the service or profession, emphasised through loyalty clauses in contracts which set limits on the freedom of staff to speak publicly. The commercialisation of health services has also placed limits on information, in that many Trust decisions are considered commercially sensitive, and therefore outside the public domain. At the same time, the amount of funding that is available for health services is firmly controlled by the state. Professional staff are compelled to consider whether a referral can be made for a patient, or a course of treatment can be afforded in a way that they have not had to do since before 1948. The need to maintain an acceptable geographical spread of emergency services sometimes cuts across the operation of the market, but there is also a potential for the operation of the market, which is most noticeable in its impact on waiting list surgery, to destabilise the operation of emergency services.

The NHS changes represent a form of post-Fordism in so far as there has been devolution of budgetary control and decision making to GP budget holders, and to the Trusts and their clinical directorates, but this is contradicted by the way that the market mechanism operates, compelling professional staff to make decisions within a tight contractual framework that is budget limited, and controlled finally by Treasury decisions. Within hospitals, the apparently contradictory principles of devolving authority to autonomous teams, and management through controlled sub-division of tasks are both evident. The language of post-Fordist autonomy that was used when the NHS reforms were introduced has recently been obscuring a process that is a modification of Taylorism. Furthermore, managerial influence over professional work is a mechanism that is likely to continue for as long as budgets are centrally determined, regardless of whether the distribution of funds is through a modified market system or based on a formula designed to secure the provision of an equitable distribution of services. Budgets are set centrally, and extra funding to any significant level cannot be drawn into the service without destroying the principle of equitable access, free at the point of acute need, that is part of the ethos of NHS care.

Doctors

Medicine has long had a form of organisation far removed from Fordism. As an ancient profession, medicine has successfully cultivated the autonomy of medical practitioners for centuries. Doctors have considerably more autonomy over their work than would be the case in a Fordist model. Doctors' individual decisions concerning patient treatment are justified in terms of clinical freedom performed in the best interests of the patient. Medicine is a highly self-regulating profession. Doctors are, once qualified, deemed to be able to deal with any situation that they consider themselves to be professionally competent to deal with. Their knowledge is seen as indeterminate, in the sense that it can never be fully written down, because of the nature of the judgement involved. The professional judgement thus cannot be subject to ordinary assessment and surveillance. Each situation to which a doctor applies his or her professional expertise is different and involves judgement as well as rules. This quality of indeterminacy, which is partly a product of complexity and variety, is sometimes seen in the literature on professions to constitute the essential trait of a profession. It is perhaps more accurately described as the basis of the successful claim to be treated as a profession. There is a significant amount of self-regarding myth in such descriptions of professionals by themselves which sociologists have repeatedly emphasised (Freidson, 1970; Johnson, 1972).

But if medicine is non-Fordist, is it post-Fordist? There are features of doctors' work style which might be described as post-Fordist, including its high level of skill combined with considerable worker autonomy, self-regulation and flexibility over tasks and working hours. However, there is an ambiguity over the relationship between doctors and their customers. While the traditional model of the doctor–patient relationship is consistent with post-Fordism, most doctors in hospitals work as part of teams and bureaucracies in ways which are far from this traditional model.

The 1990–91 changes based on the 1989 White Paper *Working for Patients* and the introduction of medical audit provide greater surveillance over the clinical freedom of individual doctors by making them open to scrutiny for medical decisions, and by more tightly specifying contracts for consultants. Ostensibly, medical audit was a matter of peer review and so did not breach the principle of doctors' clinical autonomy, but it is generally regarded as a tool with the potential to shift the balance of power between doctors and managers towards the latter. The 1990 changes also introduced new contracts for consultants which more tightly specified their work practices, for instance, that annually reviewed contracts should show a work programme for each morning and afternoon. Management concerns were to be pertinent to merit awards and general managers were to be on consultants' appointment committees. The supplement to the White Paper expressly noted that these were issues in which there was 'a need for an improved process of accountability' (Department of Health, 1989b).

Nurses

As has been shown in earlier chapters, nurses have long been subject to certain forms of control of which Henry Ford would have been proud. Despite the high level of training and expertise, and despite sometimes apparently highly autonomous working conditions, especially at night, there are many features of a Fordist regime. Nurses have to be trained and, until recently, minutely certificated. They have a rigid, bureaucratic internal hierarchy. Their conduct is rule bound and in some areas of work minor infractions are dealt with severely. They work strictly documented hours. The overall direction of their work is contested by others, doctors, who prescribe the treatment for patients. This is not unique to the UK; indeed in Canada the changing organisation of nursing, which has some similar dynamics, has been referred to as simultaneously one of professionalisation and proletarianisation (Coburn, 1988).

There is a question as to why nursing is organised in this way and whether it is the most efficient way. It is a mode of organisation which, from a post-Fordist viewpoint, under-uses the skills and capabilities of trained nurses. Nurses' capacity for informed judgement has been precluded by the demands that nurses follow tightly prescribed rules, but this is changing with the new code of practice introduced by the UKCC in 1992. While some of these rules are accepted as being consistent with good practice, there were a considerable number of instances in our study where they were reasonably perceived as being unduly rigid. The current Fordist-style governance is under considerable pressure to change.

Post-Fordist modes of governance have been recently developing in nursing. Functional flexibility has been enhanced by the three related developments mentioned above. First, Project 2000 was a major initiative which sought to upgrade nursing training. This demanded higher training standards, the inclusion of more general principles and a broader curriculum and the removal of training from hospital-led institutions to more separate provision in higher education.

Secondly, the development of primary nursing is an example of functional flexibility. Primary nursing changes the way that nurses organise their work, involving a shift from a task division of labour to a patient-centred form of care. Rather than several nurses working a ward, any of whom might do tasks for the patients, this is a system in which a nurse looks after a small group of patients largely on their own, enabling the patient to receive a more individually and sensitively tailored package of care (Salvage, 1992). There has been a grassroots movement to primary nursing, some aspects of which have been endorsed by the Patient's Charter.

A third development in summer 1992 has been the UKCC's change in its code of practice whereby nurses, once trained, are to be regarded as professionally accomplished and trusted to act within their competency, leaving behind the previous system of tightly specified and minutely certificated specialist training (UKCC, 1992b). This is a major change in the principles underlying pro-fessional practice in the issue around extended practice in nursing. It states that 'principles for practice' should replace 'certificates for tasks' as the basis of deciding adjustments to nursing practice, rejecting the traditional premise that a nurse's competence is best regulated and evidenced by certificated training. The UKCC sug-gests that the practice of 'extended' or 'extending roles' has led to the limitation of the parameters of practice preferring instead a holistic concept of nursing care. This is a change which has far-reaching implications for professionalism within nursing and repre-sents a move from a rule-focused approach to one of individual judgement, providing that it is not countermanded by individual hospitals producing their own version of an extended role system.

While there are exceptions, there is currently a general move-ment in the organisation of nursing away from Fordism in the UK. These changes are partly a result of pressure within nursing itself to become more conventionally professional. This has been aided by the changing position of women in society, and the increased access of women to higher education and training and to political influence. These processes have been supported by the apparent congruence between the nurses' project of up-skilling and greater autonomy and current political projects which prioritise the inter-ests of the consumer in issues such as more individually tailored packages of care. There is not unanimity on these changes, however. Some nurses fear that developments such as Project 2000 will lead to the creation of an elite of highly trained nurses, at the expense of the expansion of a lower rank of less trained staff, while others believe that the principles of primary nursing require all nurses to be highly trained. In some ways this debate within nursing reflects the division between Piore and Sabel's (1984) optimism about the extent of job upskilling, and Atkinson's (1986) model of a division between core and peripheral workers.

While the main impetus within registered nursing is to upgrade the training of nurses, there is also a process of change in the occupation immediately beneath it in the hospital hierarchy: the care assistants. The boundary between qualified nurses and nursing assistants is currently undergoing a major restructuring. Numerous factors are compelling a rethink of health professional/vocational boundaries and the effect is most visible at the nurse/carer boundary.

There has been the development of the NVQ system of accreditation, and related NVQ training courses; a debate on how to reduce junior doctor hours in the context of the reluctance of the nursing profession to take on some tasks from junior doctors; the removal of student nurses from the payroll of hospitals as they become supernumerary, and not part of the staffing establishment; the greater freedom that Trusts have to set their own salaries and job descriptions (not apparently yet widely used); relatively high unemployment levels, so that there is no shortage of nurses; and growing managerial interest in nursing skill-mix evaluation, as part of a way of controlling hospital costs as budget pressure intensifies even further.

Nursing's Project 2000 professionalisation strategy has left a potential hole in service provision just at the point when managerial control of hospital staffing has been extended by the introduction of Trusts, NVQs have been established, and there is a need to do something about junior doctors' tasks.

The NVQ system provides qualifications for women who otherwise would be unlikely to gain any effective qualifications because it is based around certificating skills acquired when actually at work. This is particularly important for women returners, arriving in the labour market after a period of years looking after children, who have few if any qualifications. However, it potentially undercuts the professionalisation strategy of nursing, with the creation of a pool of partially qualified health workers at significantly lower wages. The future development of this grouping may well be significant.

Ancillary workers

An increase in numerical flexibility (cf. Atkinson, 1986) in health work can be seen in the contracting out of ancillary workers, following the insistence from the mid-1980s that there should be compulsory competitive tendering for these services (Cousins, 1988;

Ham, 1992; Harrison et al., 1990; Pulkingham, 1992). This is the classic method of sub-contracting a service to another employer who is supposed to be more efficient because more specialised to that market niche, and is also able to reduce the conditions of employment, because the benefits obtained by unions are not transferred to these sub-contracted workers. The reduction in the employment rights of these workers is currently subject to challenge in the European Court.

This shift was achieved by compulsory competitive tendering (alongside that in local authorities) from 1983, when small groups of jobs were sub-contracted out, for instance, laundry services and cleaning. While in most cases in-house teams were able to win the contract, none the less it exposed these workers to the pressures of the casualised sector of the labour market. The Department of Health estimated that it saved £110m in the first year (Cousins, 1988; Ham, 1992). Cousins (1988) and Ham (1992) suggest that the net outcome was a diminution in the terms and conditions of employment of the workers, such as pay and job security, and controversy over whether the previous standards of service were maintained.

The treatment of ancillary workers in the early and mid-1980s was an example of the pessimistic version of post-Fordism with the deliberate development of a peripheral workforce with lower pay and less secure terms of service. The introduction of sub-contracting, the putting out to tender of the ancillary services, is a classic move to cut costs, and to numerical rather than functional flexibility. Under pressure to cut costs this change was to harsher conditions of employment for a more casualised workforce, risking the loss of the previous build-up of commitment among the workers. Another classic dimension of numerical flexibility was the growth of part-time work over the post-war period, as in many services, at all levels of employment and is consistent with Atkinson's model of numerical flexibility in 'peripheral' workers.

Skill, core–periphery and gender

The restructuring of health work has involved complex readjustment of not only the boundaries between doctors and nurses, but within these professions and their boundary with other workers, notably care assistants and managers. The changes in health are complex and defy easy typification in terms of the golden or pessimistic scenarios of post-Fordism. The nurses have pursued a strategy of professionalisation which may include them in the golden scenario, but simultaneously create the space for larger numbers of less qualified workers. Doctors will remain at the core and are engaged in shedding some of the more unpleasant aspects of their work, both in terms of excessive hours for juniors and the less skilled tasks, even as they lose some of their autonomy over their clinical decisions.

Health work is crucial for understanding the future of women's work and of gender relations in employment. Nurses have long been one of the best qualified groups of female workers; together with teachers they constitute the highest of the professions which are mainly female. The efforts of nurses to improve their position through a strategy of greater training and professionalisation is thus of wider interest. They have managed to make some improvements, as discussed above, both in their professional training and codes, and in ward-based competencies, though they have opened a potentially large space for lesser qualified workers, especially the NVQ qualified health care assistants. This may have an effect on the number of registered nurses employed, but at the same time there is a wider opportunity for other groups of women without formal qualifications to enter employment within health care.

The existence of nursing as a highly skilled occupation predominantly filled by women has long contradicted simple assertions that women have the least skilled jobs in the labour market, or that they are merely peripheral workers. Gender cross-cuts these developments in health work in a way not often recognised by writers on post-Fordism. All women are not being relegated to the periphery; some are. The system of employing nurses as part of a 'bank' to be drawn on when there is increased demand for nursing care is an interesting process that is not easily located in either the golden or pessimistic post-Fordism scenarios. Properly managed, the bank nursing system provides flexibility and continuity for the nurses involved as well as for their employers. Women who have access to training will be in the core; those typically older women, returning to paid work after a period of unpaid work looking after children, are more likely to be in the new periphery. Medicine is undergoing a quite dramatic change in its gender composition in entry level positions, though this effect is less marked at senior levels.

The significance of organisational structures and culture was shown by the way our respondents articulated views of their profession with no discernible differences according to their gender. That the professions are gendered is not in dispute, nor that this is related to the predominantly female one being less privileged than the predominantly male one; but there was a hegemony of the occupation over the appropriate response to the questions of conflict between the professions, despite the gender of the individual.

The drive to post-Fordism

There is a movement towards post-Fordism in NHS hospitals, but it is restricted by inadequate budgets as well as some management processes. There are differences between sections of the workforce. Doctors already had many of the features of a post-Fordist mode of governance before the introduction of markets and managers, while nurses are taking the opportunity to combine a renewed professionalisation project with a post-Fordist mode of governance. The tension between the different principles of social organisation is one of the sources of problems in interprofessional working.

The reasons for change are complex and vary between different areas of employment. Nursing is the section of the health service which has moved furthest and fastest in a post-Fordist direction in the past decade or so. This has been a change actively sought by the nurses themselves (although there are divisions in the ranks). They have pushed for improved training and education leading to a more highly skilled workforce. They face the dilemma as to whether this will lead to the Piore and Sabel (1984) version of all of them having enriched jobs, or whether they will be split into a core and periphery in the Atkinson (1986) scenario. They have led the move to a more patient-centred form of care and ward organisation. Primary nursing is a key part of the new nursing agenda (a 'bandwagon' as far as the *Nursing Times* is concerned). Nevertheless, it is reflected in government policy on the creation of named nurses.

These moves to patient-centred care are consistent with the development of consumerism in health care. This movement has had its clearest successes in the struggles by women to have birthing organised around their needs and wants, rather than those of the medical or nursing professions; and in the change in the care of children, so that parents can be with them much more in hospital. Some nursing demands are thus pushing in the same direction as the consumer movement in health care. Patients, however, have not typically had a large say in the changes in the NHS, in striking contrast to government rhetoric. Thus we would be cautious about the extent to which these changes are consumer led.

The main cause of the wider structural change has been political. The NHS was one of the least expensive health services in the West, before the introduction of markets and managers. The relations of production in health had not reached their limit of development, nor had the market for these services become saturated, contradicting Aglietta's theory. None the less, a desire to contain costs was a major reason behind the changes, even though these were not high by international standards, and even though no other model of health care organisation was cheaper. The restructuring of the NHS was politically led, based on an assumption that markets were superior to planning. The government was able to implement its proposals because it gave the opportunity to a cadre with a willingness to implement them, that is, the general managers.

The irony of the changes is that the mode of governance of medicine in its traditional professional form meets more of the requirements of new wave management and is more consistent with post-Fordism than the new structures being put into place which require Fordist-style bureaucracies to run the market. The weakness of the old system is that pre-Fordist professional autonomy was not balanced by an adequate system of monitoring and evaluation of outcomes, or adequate public accountability. While new wave management processes are clearly present within the NHS, Taylorist practices also thrive. As most management theory turns away from Taylorist models of worker behaviour, we see it being used in the NHS in order to meet the goal of cost containment. The patient is not constructed as the consumer in the new markets, and hence does not have the power of purchasing which is the basis of the progressive optimism in post-Fordist and new wave management theory alike.

In the health service today, we see nursing moving in a post-Fordist direction in terms of its internal mode of governance and its relations with its clients, but restricted in this movement by tight Fordist control at the level of hospital managers concerned with cost-containment. Cost-containment policies related to markets will force it in a Fordist direction as medicine learns to manage budgets.

In NHS hospitals we see differing degrees of Fordism, post-Fordism and pre-Fordism among the nursing and medical professions. There currently appears to be a move towards convergence, as nurses move from a near Fordist structure to a more flexible form of professionalism, while doctors' previously pre-Fordist practices also move somewhat nearer to a post-Fordist responsiveness to users through systems of audit and evaluation of outcomes. Fordist structures are limiting the move to post-Fordism because of the requirement to exercise so tight a control over costs.

The typical assumption that a move towards post-Fordism involves a greater emphasis on the consumer is problematic because of the difficulty in constructing the concept of 'consumer' where there is a separation between the purchaser and the recipient of services. When the purchaser and recipient are different it is not clear that the concept of consumer, which usually assumes these are the same, is useful. Markets and quasi-markets are not an all or nothing issue, but rather subject to a specific range of application and to various important modes of regulation. Furthermore, the possibility exists that modifications of the purchaser–provider network could develop that remove the market in health care and replace it with more stable contracts which devolve authority downwards. Patients, if not consumers, could be empowered by mechanisms other than markets, such as democracy, greater information and representation. However, the tension between the Fordist and post-Fordist modes of governance of the health professions is currently generating a form of devolved Taylorism.

Appendix

Results from hospital interviews

We are grateful to Brian Francis of the Centre for Applied Statistics at Lancaster University for carrying out the modelling.

Some interviews with medical and nursing staff could not be completed. The numbers responding to particular questions are therefore sometimes less than the total number of respondents interviewed.

Table A1 *Number of doctors and nurses reporting that they routinely work as a team (analysis by hospital and specialty)*

Specialty	Hospital					
	Greenfield ($n = 56$)	College ($n = 56$)	Central ($n = 48$)	County ($n = 45$)	City ($n = 42$)	Total per specialty
Medicine ($n = 62$)	11/20	7/12	6/13	4/9	5/8	33/62
Surgery ($n = 46$)	7/10	4/11	11/12	3/6	3/7	28/46
ENT ($n = 20$)	1/1	2/7	–	1/5	3/7	7/20
Psychiatry ($n = 29$)	8/8	–	5/8	3/7	3/6	19/29
Care of the elderly ($n = 33$)	5/8	4/5	5/8	3/6	5/6	22/33
ICU ($n = 32$)	6/6	2/7	3/7	2/5	4/7	17/32
Paediatrics ($n = 14$)	–	1/9	–	2/5	–	3/14
Theatre, A&E ($n = 11$)	3/3	2/5	–	2/2	0/1	7/11
Total per hospital	41/56	22/56	30/48	20/45	23/42	136/247

Table A2   *Number of doctors and nurses reporting no recent conflict (analysis by hospital and specialty)*

Specialty	Hospital					
	Greenfield ($n = 56$)	College ($n = 55$)	Central ($n = 49$)	County ($n = 50$)	City ($n = 50$)	Total per specialty
Medicine ($n = 63$)	12/19	1/12	2/13	4/10	6/9	25/63
Surgery ($n = 49$)	5/10	5/11	1/12	3/7	4/9	18/49
ENT ($n = 19$)	0/1	1/6	–	2/5	2/7	5/19
Psychiatry ($n = 30$)	2/8	–	3/8	1/7	2/7	8/30
Care of the elderly ($n = 37$)	5/8	3/5	1/8	2/7	2/9	13/37
ICU ($n = 36$)	3/7	1/7	2/8	0/6	2/8	8/36
Paediatrics ($n = 15$)	–	4/9	–	3/6	–	7/15
Theatre, A&E ($n = 11$)	2/3	0/5	–	0/2	1/1	3/11
Total per hospital	29/56	15/55	9/49	15/50	19/50	87/260

Bibliography

Abel-Smith, Brian (1960) *A History of the Nursing Profession*. London: Heinemann.
Abel-Smith, Brian (1984) *Cost-containment in Health Care: a Study of 12 European Countries*. Occasional Papers in Social Administration no. 73. London: Bedford Square Press/NVCO.
Abercrombie, Nicholas and Urry, John (1983) *Capital, Labour and the New Middle Classes*. London: Allen & Unwin.
Ackroyd, Stephen (1992) 'Nurses and the prospects of participative management' in Keith Soothill, Christine Henry and Kevin Kendrick (eds), *Themes and Perspectives in Nursing*. London: Chapman & Hall.
Ackroyd, Stephen, Hughes, John A. and Soothill, Keith (1989) 'Public sector services and their management', *Journal of Management Studies*, 16, 6.
Aglietta, M. (1987) *A Theory of Capitalist Regulation*. London: Verso.
Andrews, Geoff (ed.) (1991) *Citizenship*. London: Lawrence & Wishart.
Appleby, John (1992) *Financing Health Care in the 1990s*. Milton Keynes: Open University Press.
Atkinson, J. (1986) *Changing Work Patterns: How Companies Achieve Flexibility to Meet New Needs*. London; National Economic Development Office.
Audit Commission (1991) *The Virtue of Patients: Making Best Use of Ward Nursing Resources*. London: HMSO.
Bagguley, Paul, Mark-Lawson, Jane, Shapiro, Dan, Urry, John, Walby, Sylvia and Warde, Alan (1990) *Restructuring: Place, Class and Gender*. London: Sage.
Bagust, Adrian, Prescott, John and Smith, Anthony (1988) 'Numbering the nurses', *Health Services Journal*, 7 July, pp. 766–7.
Bartlett, W. and LeGrand, J. (1994) 'The performance of trusts' in R. Robinson and J. LeGrand (eds), *Evaluating the NHS Reforms*. London: King's Fund Institute.
Bell, Daniel (1973) *The Coming of Post-Industrial Society*. New York: Basic Books.
Beynon, Huw (1990) 'The miners strike'. Paper presented to BSA conference.
Bourne, Michael and Ezzamel, Mahmoud (1986) 'Organizational culture in hospitals in the National Health Service', *Financial Accountability and Management*, 2 (3): 203–25.
Bourne, Michael and Ezzamel, Mahmoud (1987) 'Budgetary devolution in the National Health Service and universities in the United Kingdom', *Financial Accountability and Management* 3 (1): 29–45.
Braverman, Harry (1974) *Labor and Monopoly Capital*. New York: Monthly Review Press.
Burrage, Michael and Torstendahl, Rolf (eds) (1990) *Professions in Theory and History: Rethinking the Study of Professions*. London: Sage.
Busfield, Joan (1990) 'Sectoral divisions in consumption: the case of medical care', *Sociology*, 24 (1): 77–96.
Butler, John (1992) *Patients, Policies and Politics: Before and After 'Working for Patients'*. Milton Keynes: Open University Press.

Carchedi, G. (1977) *On the Economic Identification of Social Classes*. London: Routledge.

Carlisle, Daloni (1991) 'Just one slip', *Nursing Times*, 87 (14): 30–1.

Carr-Hill, Roy, Dixon, Paul, Gibbs, Ian, Griffiths, Mary, Higgins, Moira, McCaughan Dorothy and Wright, Ken (1992) *Skill Mix and the Effectiveness of Nursing Care*. York: Centre for Health Economics, University of York.

Chapman, Paul (1991) 'Health care assistants', *Nursing Times*, 87 (25): 30–1.

Clarke, John and Newman, Janet (1994) 'Managerialism and the restructuring of welfare' in John Clarke, Alan Cochrane and Eugine McLaughin (eds), *Managing Social Policy*. London: Sage.

Clarke, John, Cochrane, Alan and McLaughlin, Eugine (eds) (1994) *Managing Social Policy*. London: Sage.

Coburn, David (1988) 'The development of Canadian nursing: professionalization and proletarianization', *International Journal of Health Services*, 18 (3): 437–56.

Cockburn, Cynthia (1985) *Machinery of Dominance: Women, Men and Technical Know How*. London: Pluto Press.

Cousins, Christine (1988) 'The restructuring of welfare work: the introduction of general management and the contracting out of ancillary services in the NHS', *Work Employment and Society*, 2: 210–28.

Cox, David (1992) 'Indeterminacy and technicality in health professions'. Paper presented to the BSA conference.

Crompton, Rosemary and Sanderson, Kay (1989) *Gendered Jobs and Social Change*. London: Unwin Hyman.

Dalley, G. (1993) 'The ideological foundations of informal care' in A. Kitson (ed.), *Nursing: Art and Science*. London: Chapman & Hall. pp. 11–25.

Davies, Celia (ed.) (1980) *Rewriting Nursing History*. London: Croom Helm.

Davies, Celia (1990) *The Collapse of the Conventional Career*. English Nursing Board (ENB) Project Paper 3. London: ENB.

Davis, Karen, Anderson, Gerard F., Rowland, Diane and Steinberg, Earl P. (1990) *Health Care Cost Containment*. Baltimore, MD: Johns Hopkins University Press.

Deem, Rosemary and Brehony, Kevin (1993) 'Governing bodies and local education authorities: who shall inherit the earth?', *Local Government Studies*, 19 (1): 56–76.

Denton, Miles, Morgan, Marina S. and White, Ruth R. (1991) 'Quality of prescribing of intravenous antibiotics in a district general hospital', *British Medical Journal*, 302: 327–8.

Department of Health (1988/9) *Annual Censuses of NHS Manpower, Welsh Office and Scottish Common Service Agency*. London: HMSO.

Department of Health (1989a) *Working for Patients*. White Paper, Cm 555. London: HMSO.

Department of Health (1989b) NHS Review Working Paper no. 7. *NHS Consultants: Appointments, Contracts and Distinction Awards*. London: HMSO.

Department of Health (1991a) 'William Waldegrave reassures junior doctors on pay and conditions and announces £46 million for the development of medical audit'. Press Release, 29 January. London: Department of Health.

Department of Health (1991b) *Women Doctors and their Careers*. Report of the Joint Working Party. London: Department of Health.

Department of Health (1993) *Changing Childbirth*. London: HMSO.

Department of Health and Social Security (1972) *The Second Report of the Joint Working Party on the Organisation of Medical Work in Hospitals* ('Cogwheel'). London: HMSO.

Dowling, Sue and Barrett, Sue (1991) *Doctors in the Making: the Experience of the Pre-registration Year*. Bristol: SAUS, University of Bristol.

Drucker, P.F. (1993) *The Post-capitalist Society*. Oxford: Butterworth–Heinemann.

Duncan, A.S. and McLachlan, G. (eds) (1984) *Hospital Medicine and Nursing in the 1980s: Interaction between the Professions of Medicine and Nursing*. London: Nuffield Provincial Hospital Trusts.

Edwards, Richard (1979) *Contested Terrain: the Transformation of the Workplace in the Twentieth Century*. London: Heinemann.

Edwards, Richard C., Gordon, David M. and Reich, Michael (1975) *Labor Market Segmentation*. Lexington, MA: Lexington Books.

Ehrenreich, Barbara and Ehrenreich, J. (1977) 'The professional managerial class', *Radical America* 11 (2): 12–17.

Elger, T. (1979) 'Valorisation and deskilling – a critique of Braverman', *Capital and Class*, 7: 58–99.

Elger, T. (1991) 'Task flexibility and the intensification of labour in UK manufacturing in the 1980s', in Anna Pollert (ed.), *Farewell to Flexibility?* Oxford: Blackwell.

Elston, Mary Ann (1991) 'The politics of professional power: medicine in a changing health service', in Jonathan Gabe, Michael Calnan and Michael Bury (eds), *The Sociology of the Health Service*. London: Routledge.

England, Paula (1982) 'The failure of human capital theory to explain occupational sex segregation', *Journal of Human Resources*, 17: 358–70.

Equal Opportunities Commission (1991) *Equality Management: Women's Employment in the NHS*. Manchester: EOC.

Farmer, E.S. (1989) 'Accountability at the sharp end', *Update: Nursing Board for Scotland Newsletter*, December.

Fisher, Michael (1991) 'Junior doctors and drips', *British Medical Journal*, 302: 730.

Flynn, Norman (1990) *Public Sector Management*. Hemel Hempstead: Harvester Wheatsheaf.

Flynn, Rob (1992) *Structures of Control in Health Management*. London: Routledge.

Foucault, Michel (1973) *Birth of the Clinic*. London: Tavistock.

Francis, Brian, Green, M. and Payne, C. (eds) (1993) *GLIM Manual*. Oxford: Oxford University Press.

Freeling, Paul (1986) 'Communication between doctors and nurses', in Sir John Walton and Gordon McLachlan (eds), *Partnership or Prejudice: Communication in Other Caring Professions: a Collection of Essays by a Nuffield Working Party on Communication*. London: Nuffield Provinical Hospital Trusts.

Freidson, E. (1970) *Professional Dominance: the Social Structure of Medical Care*. New York: Atherton Press.

Freidson, E. (1986) 'The medical profession in transition', in L.H. Aiken and D. Mechanic (eds), *Applications of Social Science to Clinical Medicine and Health Policy*. New Brunswick: Rutgers University Press, pp. 63–79.

Friedman, Andy (1977) 'Responsible autonomy versus direct control over the labour process', *Capital and Class*, 1: 43–57.

Friend, Bernadette (1993) 'Under fire', *Nursing Times*, 89 (18): 19.

Gamarnikow, Eva (1978) 'Sexual division of labour: the case of nursing', in Annette Kuhn and Ann-Marie Wolpe (eds), *Feminism and Materialism*. London: Routledge.

Gilligan, Carol (1982) *In a Different Voice*. Cambridge, MA: Harvard University Press.

Glennerster, Howard, Owens, Patricia and Kimberley, Angela (1986) *The Nursing*

Management Function after Griffiths: a Study of the North West Thames Region. London: London School of Economics.

Glucksmann, Miriam (1990) *Women Assemble.* London: Routledge.

Greenwood, E. (1957) 'The attributes of a profession', *Social Work* 2: 44–55.

Hakim, Catherine (1987a) 'Trends in the flexible workforce', *Employment Gazette* 95: 549–60.

Hakim, Catherine (1987b) *Home-based Work in Britain.* A report on the 1981 National Homeworking Survey and the DE Research Programme on Homework. Research Paper no. 60. London: Department of Employment.

Hall, Stuart (1988) *The Hard Road to Renewal: Thatcherism and the Crisis of the Left.* London: Verso.

Hall, Stuart and Jacques, Martin (eds) (1989) *New Times: the Changing Face of Politics in the 1990s.* London: Lawrence & Wishart.

Ham, Christopher (1992) *Health Policy in Britain: the Politics and Organisation of the National Health Service,* 3rd edn. Basingstoke: Macmillan.

Hancock, Christine (1991) 'Clinical directorates', *Nursing Standard,* 5 (24): 3–5.

Handy, Charles (1984) *The Future of Work.* Oxford: Martin Robertson.

Handy, Charles (1990) *The Age of Unreason.* London: Arrow.

Harrison, Stephen, Hunter, David and Pollitt, Christopher (1990) *The Dynamics of British Health Policy.* London: Unwin Hyman.

Harrison, Stephen, Hunter, David J., Mamoch, Gordon and Pollitt, Christopher (1992) *Just Managing: Power and Culture in the National Health Service.* Basingstoke: Macmillan.

Hartmann, Heidi (1979) 'Capitalism, patriarchy and job segregation by sex', in Zillah R. Eisenstein (ed.), *Capitalist Patriarchy.* New York: Monthly Review Press.

Haug, M. (1973) 'Deprofessionalization: an alternative hypothesis for the future', *Sociological Review,* Monograph 20: 195–211.

Health Service Management Journal (1994) Viewpoint. March, 3.

Hearn, Jeff (1982) 'Notes on patriarchy, professionalisation and the semi-professions', *Sociology,* 16 (2): 184–202.

Heyssel, R. et al. (1984) 'Decentralised management in a teaching hospital', *New England Journal of Medicine* Special Report, 310 (22): 1477–80.

Hugman, Richard (1991) *Power in Caring Professions.* Basingstoke: Macmillan.

Iglehart, J.K. (1987) 'Problems facing the nursing profession', *New England Journal of Medicine,* 317: 646–51.

Ignatieff, Michael (1991) 'Citizenship and moral narcissism', in Geoff Andrews (ed.), *Citizenship.* London: Lawrence & Wishart.

Illman, John (1991) *Guardian,* 29 September.

Jamous, H. and Peloille, B. (1970) 'Changes in the French university hospital system', in J.A. Jackson (ed.), *Professions and Professionalisation.* Cambridge: Cambridge University Press.

Jessop, Bob (1991) 'Thatcherism and flexibility: the white heat of a post-Fordist revolution', in Bob Jessop, Hans Kastendiek, Klaus Nielson and Ove K. Pedersen (eds), *The Politics of Flexibility.* Aldershot: Edward Elgar.

Jessop, Bob, Kastendiek, Hans, Nielson, Klaus and Pedersen, Ove K. (eds) (1991) *The Politics of Flexibility.* Aldershot: Edward Elgar.

Johnson, T. (1972) *Professions and Power.* London: Macmillan.

Johnson, T. (1977) 'Professions in the class structure', in Richard Scase (ed.), *Industrial Society: Class, Cleavage and Control.* London: Allen & Unwin.

Jones, G.R. (1983) 'Transaction costs, property rights and organisational culture: an exchange perspective', *Administrative Science Quarterly*, 28: 454–67.

Joule, N. (1992) 'User involvement in Medical Audit: a spoke in the wheel or a link in the chain'. London: The Greater London Association of Community Health Councils.

Kay, John and Vickers, John (1990) 'Regulatory reform: an appraisal', in Giandomenico Majone (ed.), *Deregulation or Re-Regulation? Regulatory Reform in Europe and the United States*. London: Pinter.

Kerrison, S., Packwood, T. and Buxton, M. (1994) 'Monitoring medical audit' in R. Robinson and J. LeGrand (1994) (eds) *Evaluating the NHS Reforms*. London: King's Fund Institute.

Kitson, Alison (1993) 'Formalizing concepts relating to nursing and caring', in Alison Kitson (ed.), *Nursing: Art and Science*. London: Chapman & Hall.

Klein, Rudolf (1989) *The Politics of the NHS*, 2nd edn. London: Longman.

Kocka, Jurgen (1990) ' "Burgertum" and professions in the nineteenth century: two alternative approaches', in Michael Burrage and Rolf Torstendahl (eds), *Professions in Theory and History: Rethinking the Study of Professions*. London: Sage.

Kreckel, R. (1980) 'Unequal opportunity structure and labour market segmentation', *Sociology* 4: 525–50.

Larkin, G. (1983) *Occupational Monopoly and Modern Medicine*. London: Tavistock.

Larson, M. (1977) *The Rise of Professionalism*. California: University of California Press.

Lash, S. and Urry, J. (1987) *The End of Organized Capitalism*. Cambridge: Polity.

LeGrand, Julian and Bartlett, Will (eds) (1993) *Quasi-Markets and Social Policy*. London: Macmillan.

Levitt, Ruth and Wall, A. (1992) *The Reorganised National Health Service*, 4th edn. London: Chapman & Hall.

Light, Donald (1990a) 'Learning from their mistakes', *The Health Service Journal*, 4: 1470–2.

Light, Donald (1990b) 'Bending the rules', *The Health Service Journal*, 11: 1513–15.

Light, Donald (1991) 'Observations on the NHS reforms: an American perspective', *British Medical Journal*, 303: 568–70.

Lipietz, Alain (1992) *Towards a New Economic Order: Postfordism, Ecology and Democracy*. Cambridge: Polity Press.

Longley, D. (1993) *Public Law and Health Services Accountability*. Milton Keynes: Open University Press.

Lorber, Judith (1990) 'Can women physicians ever be equal in the American medical profession?', in Judith Levy and Gary Marx (eds), *Current Research in Occupations and Professions*, 6. Los Angeles: JAI Press.

Lupton, Deborah, Donaldson, Cam and Lloyd, Peter (1991) 'Caveat emptor or blissful ignorance? Patients and the consumer is the ethos', *Social Science and Medicine*, 33 (5): 559–68.

Mackay, Lesley (1989) *Nursing a Problem*. Milton Keynes: Open University Press.

Mackay, Lesley (1992) 'Nursing and doctoring: where's the difference?', in Keith Soothill, Christine Henry and Kevin Kendrick (eds), *Themes and Perspectives in Nursing*. London: Chapman & Hall.

Mackay, Lesley (1993) *Doctors and Nurses: Working Together*. Edinburgh: Churchill Macmillan.

McKee, Martin and Lessof, Leila (1992) 'Nurse and doctor: whose task is it anyway?', in Jane Robinson, Alastair Gray and Ruth Elkan (eds), *Policy Issues in Nursing*. Buckingham: Open University Press.

McKinlay, J. and Arches, J. (1985) 'Towards the proletarianization of physicians', *International Journal of Health Services*, 15: 161–95.

McSweeney, P. (1991) 'The collapse of the conventional career', *Nursing Times*, 87 (31): 26–7.

Majone, Giandomenico (ed.) (1990) *Deregulation or Re-Regulation? Regulatory Reform in Europe and the United States*. London: Pinter.

Mallett, J. (1991) 'Shifting the focus of audit', *Health Service Journal*, 101 (41): 24–5.

Marginson, Paul (1991) 'Change and continuity in the employment structure of large companies', in Anna Pollert (ed.), *Farewell to Flexibility?* Oxford: Blackwell.

Marshall, R.D. and Spencer, R.I. (1974) 'A more efficient use of hospital beds?' *British Medical Journal*, 3: 27–30.

Massey, Doreen (1984) *Spatial Divisions of Labour: Social Structures and the Geography of Production*. London: Macmillan.

Maynard, Alan (1993) Presentation at NAHAT conference 'Marketing and the Health Service', 28 January, London.

Mincer, Jacob and Polackek, Solomon (1974) 'Family investments in human capital: earnings of women', *Journal of Political Economy*, 82 (2): S76–S108.

Moran, Michael and Wood, Bruce (1993) *States, Regulation and the Medical Profession*. Buckingham: Open University Press.

Mulgan, Geoff (1991) 'Power to the public', *Marxism Today*, May: 14–19.

Mumford, P. (1993) 'The future of the acute hospital: managing staff in hospitals', *King's Fund Newsletter*, 16(4): 4–5.

Murphy, R. (1984) 'The structures of closure: a critique and development of the theories of Weber, Collins, and Parkin', *British Journal of Sociology* 35: 547–67.

Neuberger, Julia (1993) 'The need to take views seriously', *King's Fund Newsletter*, 16 (2): 2.

Neumann, B., Sheaff, R. and Peel, V. (1990) *Costing Issues Arising from the Resource Management Initiative*. London: Department of Health.

NHS Management Enquiry (1983) *The Griffiths Report*. London: HMSO.

NHS Management Executive (1990) *NHS Trusts*. London: HMSO.

NHS Management Executive (1991) *Junior Doctors: the New Deal*. London: HMSO.

Office for Health Economics (1986) *Health: The Politician's Dilemma*. London: Office for Health Economics.

O'Higgins, Michael (1992) 'Strategic options for devolved financial management in community care'. Presentation to the Welfare State Programme Seminar Series, STICERD, London School of Economics.

Ouchi, W.G. (1980) 'Markets, bureaucracies and clans', *Administrative Science Quarterly*, 25: 129–41.

Ouchi, W.G. (1981) *Theory Z*. Reading, MA: Addison-Wesley.

Ovreteit, J. (1985) 'Medical dominance and the development of professional autonomy in physiotherapy', *Sociology of Health and Illness*, 7: 76–93.

Owens, Patricia and Glennerster, Howard (1990) *Nursing in Conflict*. London: Macmillan.

Parkin, Frank (1979) *Marxism and Class Theory: a Bourgeois Critique*. London: Tavistock.

Parry, N. and Parry, J. (1976) *The Rise of the Medical Profession*. London: Croom Helm.

Peters, Tom (1987) *Thriving on Chaos: Handbook for a Management Revolution*. London: Pan Books.

Peters, Thomas and Austin, Nancy (1986) *A Passion for Excellence: Leadership Difference*. New York: Harper Collins.

Peters, Thomas and Waterman, Robert (1982) *In Search of Excellence: Lessons from America's Best Run Companies*. New York: Harper Collins.

Piore, M. and Sabel, C. (1984) *The Second Industrial Divide*. New York: Basic Books.

Pollert, Anna (ed.) (1991) *Farewell to Flexibility?* Oxford: Blackwell.

Pulkingham, Jane (1992) 'Employment restructuring in the health service: efficiency initiatives, working practices and workforce composition', in *Work, Employment and Society*, 6 (3): 397–421.

Reverby, S. (1987) *Ordered to Care: The Dilemma of American Nursing, 1850–1945*. Cambridge: Cambridge University Press.

Robbins, Margaret (1991) 'Breaking up the blocs', *Marxism Today*, May: 30–3.

Robinson, Jane (1992) 'Introduction: beginning the study of nursing policy', in Jane Robinson, Alastair Gray and Ruth Elkan (eds), *Policy Issues in Nursing*. Milton Keynes: Open University Press.

Robinson, Jane, Gray, Alastair and Elkan, Ruth (eds) (1992) *Policy Issues in Nursing*. Milton Keynes: Open University Press.

Robinson, R. and LeGrand, J. (1994) (eds) *Evaluating the NHS Reforms*. London: King's Fund Institute.

Salmon B. (1968) *Report of the Committee on Senior Nurse Staff Structure*. London: HMSO.

Saltman, Richard B. and von Otter, Casten (1992) *Planned Markets and Public Competition: Strategic Reform In Northern European Health Systems*. Milton Keynes: Open University Press.

Salvage, Jane (1992) 'The new nursing: empowering patients or empowering nurses?', in Jane Robinson, Alastair Gray and Ruth Elkan (eds), *Policy Issues in Nursing*. Buckingham: Open University Press.

Saunders, Peter and Harris, Colin (1990) 'Privatization and the consumer', *Sociology*, 24 (1): 57–75.

Schultz, R. and Harrison, S. (1986) 'Physician autonomy in the Federal Republic of Germany, Great Britain and the United States', *International Journal of Health Planning and Management*, 2: 515–19.

Sheaf, Rod (1991) *Marketing for Health Services: a Framework for Communications, Evaluation and Total Quality Management*. Milton Keynes: Open University Press.

Seccombe, I. and Buchan, J. (1994) 'The changing role of the NHS personnel function' in R. Robinson and J. LeGrand (eds) *Evaluating the NHS Reforms*. London: King's Fund Institute.

Soothill, Keith, Henry, Christine and Kendrick, Kevin (eds) (1992) *Themes and Perspectives in Nursing*. London: Chapman & Hall.

Stacey, Margaret (1981) 'The division of labour revisited or overcoming the two Adams', in Philip Abrams, Rosemary Deem, Janet Finch and Paul Rock (eds), *Practice and Progress: British Sociology 1950–1980*. London: Allen & Unwin.

Stacey, Margaret (1988) *The Sociology of Health and Healing*. London: Unwin Hyman.

Standing Committee on Postgraduate Medical Education (SCOPME) (1991)

Improving the Experience: Good Practice in Senior House Officer Training: A Report on Local Initiatives. London: SCOPME.

Standing Committee on Postgraduate Medical Education (SCOPME) (1992) *Third Report*. London: SCOPME.

Standing, Guy (1989) 'Global feminization through flexible labour', *World Development*, 17 (7): 1077–95.

Strong, Philip and Robinson, Jane (1990) *The NHS – Under New Management*. Milton Keynes: Open University Press.

Sweeney, Phil (1991) 'The collapse of the conventional career', *Nursing Times*, 87 (31): 26–7.

Teeling Smith, G. (ed.) (1984) *A New NHS Act for 1996?*. London: Office for Health Economics.

UKCC (1986) *Project 2000: a New Preparation for Practice*. London: UKCC.

UKCC (1992a) 'Important announcements by the council'. Letter from UKCC Registrar and Chief Executive to all registered nurses. London: UKCC.

UKCC (1992b) *Code of Practice*, 3rd edn. London: UKCC.

UKCC (1992c) *The Scope of Professional Practice*. London: UKCC.

UKCC (1993a) *Standards for Records and Record Keeping*. London: UKCC.

UKCC (1993b) *Register*. London: UKCC.

Vollmer, H.M. and Mills, D.L. (1966) *Professionalisation*. Englewood Cliffs, NJ: Prentice Hall.

Walby, Sylvia (ed.) (1985) *Gender Segregation at Work*. Milton Keynes: Open University Press.

Walby, Sylvia (1986) *Patriarchy at Work*. Cambridge: Polity Press.

Walby, Sylvia (1989) 'Flexibility and the sexual division of labour', in Stephen Wood (ed.), *The Transformation of Work?* London: Unwin Hyman.

Walby, Sylvia (1990) *Theorising Patriarchy*. Oxford: Blackwell.

Walker, Alison (1991) 'Teaching junior doctors practical procedures', *British Medical Journal*, 302: 306.

Walton, Sir John and McLachlan, Gordon (eds) (1986) *Partnership or Prejudice: Communication in other Caring Professions: a Collection of Essays by a Nuffield Working Party on Communication*. London: Nuffield Provincial Hospital Trust.

Wandelt, M. and Ager, J. (1974) *Quality of Patient Care Scale*. New York: Appleton-Century-Crofts.

Watkins, Steve (1987) *Medicine and Labour: the Politics of a Profession*. London: Lawrence & Wishart.

Whittington, Richard (1991) 'The fragmentation of industrial R & D', in Anna Pollert (ed.), *Farewell to Flexibility?* Oxford: Blackwell.

Wilkins, A.L. and Ouchi, W.G. (1983) 'Efficient cultures: exploring the relationship between culture and organisational performance', *Administrative Science Quarterly*, 28: 468–81.

Williamson, Charlotte (1992) *Whose Standards? Consumer and Professional Standards in Health Care*. Milton Keynes: Open University Press.

Witz, Anne (1992) *Professions and Patriarchy*. London: Routledge.

Wood, Stephen (1989) 'New wave management?', *Work, Employment and Society*, 3 (3): 379–402.

Work, Employment and Society (1992). Special issue on 'Women, flexibility and the service sector', 6 (3).

Wright, Steve (1992) 'The named nurse', *Nursing Times*, 88 (11): 27–9.

Yates, John (1982) *Hospital Beds: a Problem for Diagnosis and Management*. London: Heinemann.

Index